TRAUMA
in
PERSONALITY
DISORDER

TRAUMA
in
PERSONALITY
DISORDER

A Clinician's Handbook
The Masterson Approach

Candace Orcutt, PhD

authorHOUSE®

AuthorHouse™
1663 Liberty Drive
Bloomington, IN 47403
www.authorhouse.com
Phone: 1-800-839-8640

Published by AuthorHouse   03/21/2012

ISBN: 978-1-4685-5805-0 (sc)
ISBN: 978-1-4685-5814-2 (e)

Library of Congress Control Number: 2012903635

CONTENTS

FOREWORD

The treatment of trauma in personality disorders often falls between two stools: the therapist either focuses solely on the psychic trauma overlooking the personality disorder, or focuses on the personality disorder overlooking the trauma. There is a great need in the literature for a book that focuses on the necessity to balance character work with trauma work. Dr. Orcutt's book fills this need.

Dr. Orcutt has immersed herself in the study and treatment of these disorders, and in this volume she has distilled and shared her wisdom with us.

This book, well organized and beautifully written, is unique in the degree to which it takes us into Dr. Orcutt's office and vividly and often movingly describes in detail the one to one interventions with the patient. She delineates clearly when, why, and how she shifts her intervention from trauma to the personality disorders. She presents clearly the difference between a recent trauma and an early "developmental" trauma, and how one can precipitate the other. The ebb and flow of the work between personality disorder and trauma becomes clinically clear to the reader.

The book is a must reading for all clinicians who are dealing with the therapeutic challenges of trauma and the personality disorders.

James F. Masterson, M

ACKNOWLEDGMENTS

I owe more than I can list to colleagues, patients, and friends, whose insights have gone into the building of this book. Nevertheless, certain individuals have offered so much that their names come immediately to mind and recognition. James F. Masterson, M.D., my mentor of many years, encouraged me to write this book, and reviewed its contents. Louise Gaston, Ph.D, shared her expert knowledge of trauma with me, and supported my synthesis of trauma work and character work. Patricia A. Graham, CSW, contributed her knowledge and perceptive insights. Alice Watson Schell, M.A., reviewed the manuscript with a writer's eye. Others who contributed their good discussion and ideas are Anne Lieberman, M.S.W., Sheila Margiotta, Ph.D., Judith Pearson, Ph.D., and Steven Reed, Ph.D. My thanks to all.

AUTHOR'S NOTE

The case illustrations given in Section II are composites. I have chosen to present cases in this form in order to preserve patient anonymity, and to include as many typical elements as possible in a single case example. I hope that this inclusiveness will make the cases as informative as possible, while preserving the liveliness of the numerous clients from whom they are drawn. On the other hand, such condensed cases, focused on teaching, have an inevitable tendency to seem oversimplified, even a little too easy, to do justice to the tangents and muddles produced during the therapeutic process by patient and therapist alike. Beyond that, an additional oversimplification comes when the telling of cases is abridged in time.

The work with personality disorders, and especially those complicated by trauma, requires enormous patience and time. The repetitive reactions of the personality disorders require repetitive interventions; work with traumatic reactions, require the same. Much effort is spent regaining ground that was already gained, then partially lost, and may be lost again before it is finally secured. This can be reflected only in part in a practical retelling.

Candace Orcutt, Ph.D

CHAPTER 1

INTRODUCTION

Psychotherapy, so rich in its theories and approaches, presents special challenges in patients' personality disorders and traumatic experiences. Clinicians trained in character work often miss the interweaving of trauma and the self, and set traumatic material aside as "crisis work" to be handled by another clinician or by medication.

On the other hand, clinicians trained in trauma techniques may not take the time, nor have the training, to deal with the characterological implications that need patience and the building of relationship to heal. The clinician trained to sit back and say little is likely to have difficulty with the more active trauma techniques (hypnosis, EMDR).

Conversely, the more active, goal-oriented clinician may be impatient with the slower, relation-building approach. This division in the field plays into the patient's pathological need to deny the management of trauma as a responsibility of the self. This kind of patient needs an approach that combines the strengthening of the self with the overcoming of trauma.

This book presents a clinical approach which balances character work with trauma work in the patient suffering from both personality disorder and trauma.

The opening section presents introductory theory and clinical information. The main section concerned with clinical application, consists of process accounts of four major types of personality disorder:

- borderline;
- manifest narcissistic;
- "closet" or hidden narcissistic;
- and schizoid.

This treatment is based on the developmental, object relations approach developed by James F. Masterson, M.D., which provides a clear theoretical base leading to specific techniques. Each case also presents a mixture of personality disorder and various forms of trauma or PTSD symptoms.

The psychotherapy of these co-existing conditions is told in casebook form to demonstrate how the therapist must keep character work and trauma work in balance during the course of treatment. The closing section deals with special issues that extend or clarify the core of the book.

"Character work" is a term generally used to describe clinical psychoanalytic psychotherapy of the disorders of the self. Originally, it was applied to maladaptive "traits" and "armoring" of the self, but widened its meaning as the field became increasingly concerned with what it came to call personality disorders—disturbances in the basic structure of the self. Here, "character work" is used in its ʌllest definition.

"Trauma work" is a term just coming into use, as the ᴐt of trauma has made its way into accepted use in the field. It addresses the major pressure placed on the integrity of the self by deeply threatening happenings that may occur at any time in life (from childhood abuse to shell shock).

Throughout the twentieth century, character work and trauma work have devolved dynamically. Character work has grown along with the development of psychoanalytic psychotherapy, which added ego psychology and object relations to a deepening concept of the self. Trauma work has grown through the increasing public and professional awareness of the impact on the individual of violence, whether accidental (plane crashes), familial (domestic violence, incest), or global (war and revolution).

This progress is welcome for patients suffering from either personality disorder or trauma. But in a great many patients these conditions are co-morbid, and require a balance of approaches to meet the entire problem.

Balancing character work and trauma work is a therapeutic challenge for a number of reasons. As previously mentioned: 1) training and perhaps personal predilection in the clinician may divide character work and trauma work; 2) the patient's pathology will strive to keep trauma encapsulated, and characterological issues separate and denied.

Even when character work and trauma work are united in one therapy, the divisiveness may persist. The therapist may deal well with material relating to personality in general, but shies away from ugly traumatic material (especially the more expressive—or abreactive—it gets).

Or the therapist may deal well with trauma, and be well-versed in special techniques such as hypnosis, EMDR or Thought Field Therapy, but may distance from patient's protracted need for character work. Of course patient's tendency to defensively divide the self may echo or provoke this division in the therapist. There have been attempts to bridge the gap. Mardi Horowitz has written of trauma work with a narcissistic personality. Francine Shapiro's EMDR emphasizes the need for a "cognitive interweave" to integrate sessions.

But the clinical tendency remains to push it all back (or send it elsewhere), or encourage it to all hang out—both at the expense of the patient's requirement for wholeness and process. For it is the whole, emotionally maturing patient who is the focus here.

Medicine has gained much knowledge by examining the human being in sections. But scientific knowledge (though it may lead to it) is not healing, and the more we learn about the pieces of ourselves, the more we become aware of their interdependency.

Psychotherapy—the treatment of the psyche—has as its definition the healing of the soul, or self. So clinicians have set ourselves the considerable goal of healing the whole self with every wise approach we can absorb. This sets a daunting challenge for the clinician. Not only must we learn more, we must become more. Our knowledge of theory and technique is critical for our patients' healing. But I am not sure that most patients will become more whole unless the wholeness of the therapist allows it.

Ours is a trade where professional and personal growths are intertwined. I hope that this book will encourage this process, and further enhance the interpersonal give and take of healing shared by clinician and patient.

CHAPTER 2

OVERVIEW

2.1. Overview of Theory

This book focuses on character pathology when it is mingled with traumatic experience occurring in the formative years. The trauma consists of physical and sexual abuse, which I will refer to as "developmental trauma." This early condition, usually has a profound effect on a person's life, but is nevertheless notably resistant to psychotherapy, especially since the "memory" of the experience may not be held in conscious awareness.

Two happenings, in particular, may bring this early condition to the foreground: 1) a trigger in present time, often a traumatic event; 2) the resolution of the character pathology, which apparently strengthens the self to tolerate the evolving knowledge of developmental trauma.

The person with ingrained character problems—who meets life with a limited perspective, and more or less inflexible ways of managing relationships, work, and even recreation—is unable to make adequate use of his or her energy. Energy that should be directed to an immediate concern is deflected, inhibited, or over-expended in pursuit through anxiety and depression to the desired goal, people do not pursue their intentions freely. They wander off on tangents, are stuck in procrastination, or achieve at the expense of disproportionate stress.

The self cannot call spontaneous and flexible energy into play: with a toolbox of capacities at hand, the self repeatedly uses only a file, pliers, or a hammer for every task that comes along. The self, therefore, is poorly equipped to meet the requirements of the ordinary situation, let alone the pressures of extraordinary stress.

What happens, then, when the characterologically limited self must meet the impact of trauma? Trauma also rigidifies the person's reaction to life – thoughts, feelings, issues, people are guarded against or avoided if they trigger recall of a traumatic event. Or the subject is pursued by unstoppable recollections—images, sounds, smells, tastes, sensations; repetitive thoughts and overwhelming feelings—that crowd out peace of mind in present time.

This may lead to more avoidance or aggressive behavior, even daredevil behavior, to overcome fear with risk, and to gain a false sense of control. The avoidance, denial, and aggressive and risk-taking behavior of trauma survivors may mimic maladaptive character defenses. A fearful victim stance or a stance of bullying or bravado may resemble character patterns ingrained from early life. Of course, when similar defenses and patterns exist as a result of both character pathology and trauma, the result is intensified.

Even this simplified view of the situation shows how the combination of traumatic experience and pre-existing character pathology creates a complex and intensified situation. In psychotherapy, diagnosis and treatment must efully differentiate and address overlapping conditions may duplicate and intensify each other, and certainly stubborn, resistant states.

The intertwining of traumatic stress issues and issues of character structure has been addressed to some degree in the literature. Bennett Braun (1986) stresses the importance of a secure character structure as a support for trauma work:

"Gathering facts or emotions is useless if they cannot be integrated. Abreaction, without cognitive structure can be dangerous . . . because it can activate traumatic memories for which the patient has no defense or coping skill. This in turn can lead to an escalation of acting-out behavior and psychological or physical collapse" (p. 14).

Mardi Horowitz (1997) is more explicitly concerned with how traumatic experiences "become incorporated into self schemata and concepts of relationship of self to the world" (p. 49). He presents process interviews showing the use of character-aware cognitive interventions with traumatically stressed narcissistic personality disorder.

Bessel van der Kolk, *et al.,* (1996) take up the controversial theme of the relationship between trauma and character, holding that childhood trauma has a direct causative effect on the etiology of borderline personality disorder (pp. 201-202).

Daniel Brown (1997), on the other hand, has made a clear distinction between formation of personality disorder through the mechanisms of interpersonal attachment in the formative years, and the distortions of perception and cognition imposed upon the self by discrete or intermittent experiences of trauma, even at an early age. Allan Schore (1999) is in agreement with Brown, although he sees a type of trauma mechanism influencing the brain in either case.

What emerges from sometimes conflicting statements is the likelihood of some sort of resemblance or connectedne between character pattern and the patterning effec trauma on the self.

My view is that personality disorder and the effects of developmental trauma create a comorbid condition that probably has essentially different causes, although these causes have a mutual influence upon each other. This conceptualization has a direct, significant impact on technique, as I will propose that treatment (except in acute phases) must give priority to the containing capacy of character work, while maintaining the flexibility to shift to trauma work, when trauma-related emotional pain or abreactions of traumatic experience press the patient. A duality of approach needs to be observed within a unified, prioritized technique.

2.1.1. Personality Disorder

Personality is defined in the *Diagnostic and Statistical Manual* of the American Psychiatric Association (1994) as "enduring patterns of perceiving, relating to, and thinking about the environment and oneself." *DSM-IV* continues:

> Personality traits are prominent aspects of personality that are exhibited in a wide range of personal and social contexts. Only when personality traits are inflexible and maladaptive and cause either significant functional impairment or subjective distress do they constitute a Personality Disorder. (p. 770).

This basic definition overarches the various subtypes of personality disorder discussed in the following clinical apters.

I would only emphasize that the inflexibility and daptability of personality disorder emerges from distortion in the "enduring patterns of perceiving, relating to, and thinking about . . ." that amounts to a fundamental belief system, guarded by emotion that governs attitude and behavior without conscious questioning.

I will use the terms "character" and "personality" interchangeably, although technically, the latter is an evolution of the former. This widely defined and explored subject does not require an extensive review here, although I will provide a general summary of its history, and a more detailed explanation of James Masterson, M.D.'s, developmental, self, and object relations approach to its theoretical and clinical dimensions.

The history of dynamic psychotherapy has always shown a shifting relationship—usually interactional—between the concepts of fixation and regression. Freud initiated this dichotomy, and his works reflect evolving theories of relationship between the two in psychopathology (Laplanche &. Pontalis, 1973, pp. 162-163).

In the course of Freud's work (1908), fixation gathers significance (pp. 45ff.) He includes descriptions of various "characters" whose neuroses rest more on traits and patterns of behavior than on symptomatology (1915, pp. 318ff.).

Fenichel (1945) stresses the complementarity of fixation and regression: "The more intense the pregenital fixations, the weaker the subsequent [psychic] organization."

An individual fixed on the anal level will advance only with reluctance . . . , and he will always be prepared to relinquish his new acquision upon slight disappointment or threat" (p. 160). Fenichel's increased emphasis on the importance of fixation and "character neurosis" continues the shift toward character as a central consideration psychoanalytic theory.

It is probably Wilhelm Reich, (1949) whose concept of "character armor" shifts theoretical attention significantly to the importance of character pattern. Although he continues to work with the libidinal model, his emphasis on defense supports the concept of fixations of the ego that moves to center stage with the evolving of ego psychology.

With the ascendancy of ego psychology, "fixation" of the libido gives way in primacy to forms of "ego modification," such as ego defect, ego deviation, ego distortion, and ego regression (Blanck and Blanck, 1974, pp. 92-93). The structure of the personality becomes central to the process of diagnosis:

"Diagnosis is to be made, not from the symptom or symptom cluster, but from Appraisal of the structure of the ego in which the symptom is embedded" (p. 92).

The immensely complex fields of object relations theory and developmental studies continue to shift emphasis onto personality or character patterning, each stressing (in numerous different ways with widely varying emphases) the importance of the mother-child relationship in the formation of this structuring, and how relationship is made, reciprocated, and internalized by the psyche. Bowlby (1988) describes this patterning:

"Observations lead us to conclude that toward the end of the first year of life children are acquiring considerable knowledge of their immediate world and that during subsequent years this knowledge is best regarded as becoming organized in the form of internal working models, including models of self and mother.

"Because these models are in constant use, day in and day out, their influence on thought, feeling, and behavior comes routine and largely outside of awareness (p. 4). he patterning of our way of being with ourselves and others has gradually become the predominating way we view the pathology of personality disorder (for the purposes of this book, the terms "personality" and "character" are used interchangeably).

The Diagnostic and Statistical Manual of Mental Disorders (1994) presents these patterns descriptively, viewing the patient from an objective external stance at the expense of a dynamic, though perhaps more metaphoric attitude.

In this book, I will present the dynamically-oriented developmental, self, and object relations conceptualization of personality disorder put forward by James F. Masterson, M.D. This approach goes beyond the descriptive to the more speculative, and is valued by me for two main reasons: 1) it synthesizes the more predominant and durable models of the mind; 2) it offers a theoretical base that translates into an effective clinical way of working.

2.1.2. The Developmental, Self, and Object Relations Approach

Theoretically, this approach retains the balance between fixation and regression, as did the original concept of character disorder, only the regression is brought about by separation/individuation stress, while the fixation point represents an arrest in ego development. Since personality disorder is seen as a pre-Oedipal condition, regression from Oedipal anxieties is not a major focus of therapy. The approach adds layerings of ego psychology, developmental, object relations, and self theory to the libidinal model, extending and transforming it in the process to define an inclusive view of personality disorder.

Masterson (1976, 1981) maintains the key concept transference, repetition, resistance, defense, fixation regression from Freud's original thought. These concepts are somewhat altered to maintain a focus on character/personality disorder rather than on neurotic character traits centered on Oedipal issues. The pre-Oedipal emphasis is maintained throughout.

Transference acting out, seen through the lens of early internalized object relations, is not a distortion of a whole-person perception of the other; it becomes a massive misperception of the other, which finds expression in an interpersonal response unqualified by reality-testing or ability to entertain mixed good and bad perceptions.

The *repetition compulsion* also takes on an uncompromising, avoidant nature, obeying a stereotyped definition of self, other, and relationship that arises from an inner conviction that is not influenced by objective observation of the outside world.

Resistance takes its coloration from early life, and sets its wall against changes in the self that would allow conscious awareness of issues related to separation and individuation.

The *defenses* used are also the externalizing defenses of the pre-Oedipal years: detachment, idealization, devaluation, clinging, avoidance, denial, projection, projective identification, acting out, and splitting. As previously mentioned, *fixation* becomes a developmental failure of the ego, while *regression* is triggered by the primitive anxieties of separation and individuation.

I have already noted that Masterson takes from ego psychology the concept of early *developmental arrest.* This concept intertwines with the developmental studies of Margaret Mahler, Bowlby, Stern, and Schore to conclude that developmental arrest in certain stages of ʼy child development gives a unique stamp to types ʼrsonality disorder. Thus, although arrest in the separation-individuation phase of development may lead to personality disorder, arrest in the practicing sub-phase is specific to narcissistic personality disorder, while arrest in the rapprochement sub-phase may foreshadow borderline personality disorder.

The concept from Anna Freud (1966) that defenses mature with the growing psyche is also important to Mastersonian theory, which stresses work with early defenses to prepare the way for emergence of the more sophisticated defenses of sublimation and creativity.

The importance of object relations theory to the Masterson approach has been touched upon. Internalized object relations constitute the way we take in the nature of the definition of self, other, and relationship in our early years, and use this template or program by which to gauge the relationships of our later years.

In the healthily growing child, internalized object relations mature steadily from partial perceptions into whole and flexible interworking gestalts. In personality disorder, the perception of relationship narrows and tightens not only to an immature level, but to a level that is distorted, as well.

Especially, the concepts of good and bad are isolated from each other, so that the capacity to see people and their interactions as a complex mingling of positive and negative intentions and acts is significantly compromised.

Finally, Mastersonian theory encompasses the overarching concept of the *self* (1985), which can give the perception of one's own entity its wholeness, independence, creativity, and capacity for intimacy with another.

Mastersonian theory synthesizes the primary models of the mind into a unique conceptualization that lends it to a clinical approach. The key to this application is a p

Mastersonian concept: the *disorders of the self triad,* or *separation-individuation (self activation) leads to separation anxiety and abandonment depression, which lead to the reestablishment of pre-Oedipal defense.* Spelled out, the triad describes a pathological process in the individual whose personality disorder arises from an early developmental arrest, and who may even pursue a high-functioning life until faced with a significant issue involving separation or individuation. This stressor acts as a cue to call up early feelings of depression and anxiety, which are then defended against by the same early defenses resorted to at the time of the initial arrest.

An especially virulent aspect of the triad is the pathological reversal of values that it involves. Not only does the individual regress under pressure to an earlier stage of emotional development, but the meanings of "good" and "bad" are essentially reversed.

To be healthily individuative has been met with disapproval and therefore evokes "bad'" feelings. To succumb to a conciliatory, victimized stance has been met with approval, and therefore feels "good."

"Good" and "bad" have been reversed from the healthy norm, and their definition has been modified to be nearly synonymous with "obedient" and "disobedient."

As a result of these redefinitions, as well as the fixation and regression of the triad, the clinical work with personality disorder becomes more complex than the simple undoing of an arrest through reality testing and behavioral modification. Intense feelings guard any questioning of the pathological situation, and repel attempts to understand its nature.

These feelings have been formed around childhood erience and need, and support a belief system that is protected with intensity, as it (distortedly) represents a way of surviving.

2.1.3. Trauma and PTSD

Scientific interest in traumatic stress began in the late 1800's, emerging from an intersection of the new pursuits of neurology, psychology, and sociology. The two great contributors who shaped the first major "debate" on this always-controversial subject were the French psychiatrist, Pierre Janet, and the Viennese neurologist, Sigmund Freud.

Janet reasoned that the subject of traumatic experience was unable to find expression of this experience in conscious, narrative memory; the expression was blocked by a process Janet called "dissociation" (van der Kolk et al., 1996, p.52). Janet hypothesized that the basis for dissociation was a genetic weakness—a pathological predisposition rather than a protective mechanism.

Freud, who learned much from Janet, nevertheless concluded that the "traumatic neuroses" arose from a defensive activity of the psyche, aimed at "repressing" the memory of experiences too overwhelming to be allowed to remain in the conscious domain (Orcutt, 1995, pp. 190-192).

Initially, he hypothesized that the repressed experience was one of sexual abuse in early childhood. In effect, he took the onus off the traumatized individual and placed it on society. This perceived assault on the sanctity of the family was met with profound professional disapproval. Freud eventually relinquished his "seduction theory," shifting his inquiry to inner fantasy—and, coincidentally, back onto the traumatized individual. Freud stood by his concept of unconscious defensive processes, but surrendered his socially-focused trauma concept.

The connection of so many psychically traumatic experiences to socially elevated institutions has led to a formidable social resistance to their exploration, even in scientific circles. To look at child abuse and domestic violence is to question the family system. To look at the psychic wounds of war veterans questions the idealization of the military. The institutions of the family and the military are mainstays of communal security as we know it, and our need to protect them from scrutiny has competed with our need to explore their nature in order to continually advance our civilization.

Judith Herman (1992) sketches the conflictual history of trauma research:

> The subject evokes such intense controversy that it periodically becomes anathema. Study of psychological trauma has repeatedly led into realms of the unthinkable and foundered on fundamental questions of belief (p. 7).

She demonstrates how socio-political movements bring the issue of psychic trauma into cultural awareness and repeatedly meet with a backlash. At the time of the writing of this book, the forces for once are in sufficient balance to bring this conflict itself into the open. Widespread media give a voice to the victims of trauma as well as to the opposition in a great many instances. With modern communications and the formidable grass-roots movements that speak for such groups as victimized women and abused children, it is becoming more difficult for us to culturally dissociate ourselves from the reality of psychic trauma.

Contemporary hypothesizing uses Janet's concept of dissociation and Freud's ideas of the unconscious and defense, and seeks the neurological basis of these phenomena with scientific tools not available one hundred years ago. It appears that sophisticated technology will give us the capacity to explore the nature of trauma in a pragmatic way that can turn back social denial still further.

In the process of defining trauma, the *Diagnostic and Statistical Manual* of the American Psychiatric Association has demonstrated the historical unevenness associated with this subject. As a result of the traumatic events of the second world war—widescale combat, civilian bombings, concentration camps—*DSM*-I, in 1952, included the diagnosis of "gross stress reaction." However, peacetime apparently led to the elimination of the category in *DSM-II*. Again, the experiences of Vietnam veterans brought a return of the issue of trauma as an anxiety disorder in *DSM-III* in 1980. In 1987, *DSM-III-R* made yet another revision: the accumulation of formal research and the impetus of a strong grass-roots movement concerned with war veterans, domestic violence, the rights of women and the issue of child abuse led to the defining of a specialized anxiety disorder called Post Traumatic Stress Disorder (PTSD). *DSM-IV* (1994) retained the category as Posttraumatic Stress Disorder.

D*SM-IV* defines PTSD as follows:

> The essential feature of Posttraumatic Stress Disorder is the development of characteristic symptoms following exposure to an extreme traumatic stressor involving direct personal experience of an event that involves actual or

> threatened death or serious injury, or other threat to one's physical integrity; or witnessing an event that involves death, injury, or a threat to the physical integrity of another person; or learning about expected or violent death, serious harm, or threat of death or injury experienced by a family member or other close associate . . . The person's response to the event must involve intense fear, helplessness, or horror . . . (p.424)

The diagnostic criteria for PTSD are as follows:

A. The person experienced, witnessed, or was confronted with an event or events that involved actual or threatened death or serious injury, or a threat to the physical integrity of the self or others . . .

B. The traumatic event is persistently re-experienced . . .

C. Persistent avoidance of stimuli associated with the trauma and numbing of general responsiveness . . .

D. Persistent symptoms of increased arousal . . .

E. Duration of the disturbance . . . is more than 1 month . . .

F. The disturbance causes clinically significant distress or impairment in social, occupational, or other important areas of functioning . . . (pp. 427-429)

This *DSM-IV* definition of PTSD is descriptive and generalized. Since it is theoretical, as well, it provides a working definition that receives enough consensual validation among a wide range of clinicians to make it useful as a touchstone (if not a cornerstone) for conceptualizing work with patients.

Terms such as "trauma" and "PTSD" are used here to label the impact of overwhelming external events on the inner psyche. Although this form of stress may possibly originate with a blow to the body, as Wilson (1989) says: "traumatic events occur inside the psyche of individuals" (p. 5).

2.1.4. Character and Psychic Trauma

It is interesting to note that Freud's initial formulation of hysteria is basic to both a theory of psychic trauma and a theory of pathological character formation. The key concept lies in the idea that repetitive, stereotyped behavior substitutes for memory and feeling. In Freud's early work (Breuer and Freud, 1895), psychopathology is considered to be trauma-based.

Under hypnosis and through abreaction, by joining behavior with words and feeling, traumatic experience is transformed into conscious memory and released from repetition. Later, Freud (1914) still maintained the concept of changing behavior into conscious memory, but placed this process within the context of an evolving relationship between analyst and analysand, (366ff.).

Through the free associations of the analysand and the evenly-hovering attention of the analyst, the transference emerges. The transference is then worked through to conscious awareness via the interpretations of the analyst. The trauma-based concept of transforming behavior into memory through combined words and feeling remains, but is placed within a character-based framework: the therapeutic relationship.

The tendency is to see the cathartic (abreactive) and interpretive (transference-based) approaches as antagonistic, as Freud did (in the one striking instance where he abandoned his dialectical style of thought).

But it seems to me that both approaches have to be used cooperatively while working with the traumatized patient who also suffers from personality disorder. The central theme of this book is that such patients must receive a specialized treatment for their traumatic state, but that this trauma work must be consistently contained within the relationship-based work with character.

This book focuses on disorder of personality (or character) and trauma when they originate together in the developmental years (PTSD, of course, can occur at any age). This early time of origin determines the near-inseparability of this type of co-morbidity. According to brain researchers, there is an early type of memory-described as "implicit" or "behavioral" memory-that is the predominating form of memory until around the age of three, when "narrative," or "verbal" memory takes the ascendancy (Brown, Scheflin, and Hammond, 1998. pp. 89-90).

This form of memory preserves experience in images, sensations, moods, and behaviors, but not in conscious, narrative statements and concepts. "Explicit," or "narrative" memory begins to take the lead from around three years of age, allowing the child to connect his sensations and observations with words, thus creating a story-line that organizes and communicates experience.

Implicit memory continues to exist in tandem with behavioral memory throughout life, and it is probably in implicit memory that traumatic experience is "frozen"—unable to process into the narrative flow of memory because (one hypothesizes) some "fail safe" neurological mechanism has shut down the transfer of overwhelming input into conscious awareness. The traumatized person suffers from intrusive feelings, sensations, images, and repetitive behaviors which can only be resolved by their integration and expression in full, narrative consciousness.

Personality disorder, which is shaped in these early, formative years before three, also is held in implicit, behavioral memory, and expresses itself in repetitive, maladaptive behavior.

As Freud (Breuer and Freud, 1895) might have said, the capacity to consciously verbalize, feel, and remember has been "strangulated" (p. 52).

To extend this argument: both early trauma in the developmental years and personality disorder come into being when implicit memory is ascendant, and express themselves in repeated behavioral patterns that cannot resolve themselves because they cannot find their way into words. Further, the way into words appears, in both cases, to be stopped by an emotional block that appears, on some level, to be intolerable (i.e.: traumatic experience and the abandonment depression).

In short, it would appear that the concept of the repetition compulsion is intrinsic to both personality disorder and developmental trauma—it is the unsuccessful (and therefore avoidant) attempt of the self to express the non-verbal through behavior, mood, sensation, and to fail for lack of words.

In the case of personality disorder, it is the mother-child misattunement that creates the dilemma. In the case of developmental trauma, the threat comes as an added element, whether it is based on a situation originating from outside the mother-child dyad, or on a cruel complication of the mother-child misattunement.

Although character formation and abuse appear to be processed somewhat differently, they are experienced as close in nature to each other, and are perceived as interconnected. Because of the child's early perception of the mother-child dyad as all-encompassing, developmental trauma will be understood as somehow intrinsic to the relationship, however the experience may originate. The trauma will appear to have been somehow a part of that relationship, and so attaches to it.

It is interesting to note that a persistent traumatic reaction (PTSD) in the adult years involves partial or incomplete implicit memory of a traumatic event, even though conscious memory may be painfully present in flashbacks or intrusive recollections. As a result, PTSD occurring after the formative years has somewhat less of a tendency to disguise itself in behavioral patterns. Even though these patterns (such as avoidance or risk-taking) may be present, they may appear quite separately from the patterning of the person's character style. Of course, there are frequent instances when adult trauma triggers early developmental trauma. This is an important clinical issue, but it does not essentially change the distinction between developmental trauma and PTSD acquired in later years.

The intertwining and similar behavioral patterning of personality disorder and developmental trauma present a complicated human phenomenon. The clinical implications, discussed in the next chapter, are also complex, but this book hopes to map out a theoretically feasible and practically useful clinical approach to the problem.

2.2. Overview of Clinical Technique

When personality disorder and trauma co-exist in the individual, the treatment is undeniably complex. However, the therapy focuses on certain fundamental and consistent steps. Briefly listed, these are the steps:

- Functioning
- Containment
- Strengthening
  - balance
  - pacing
  - consolidation
- Cognitive and behavioral change (shorter-term therapy)
- Insightful and dynamic change (long-term therapy)

The model of treatment I will propose is one that applies to developmental trauma (trauma occurring within the first three years of life), when adult posttraumatic stress disorder may be superimposed on early traumatic experience. This entrenched form of traumatic stress is combined with personality disorder. This model of treatment assumes that the exclusive or primary mode of therapy is outpatient.

2.2.1 The Steps of Therapy

- **Step 1: Functioning**

The patient must be able to maintain practical independence throughout this difficult work. This means there must be at least a subsistence income (including means of payment for therapy); housing and food must be assured, and some form of social network should exist, even though it may be provided by professionals and agencies. The need for this fundamental level of support cannot be stressed enough—for the security of the patient, the therapy, and the therapist.

The demands of the work are secondary to the demands of basic survival, which is threatened if (for example) the pressure of emotion evoked by character work touches off defensive acting out, or the trauma work leads to a dissociative state that interferes with the ability to hold a job.

The patient's surrounding circumstances must offer a sufficient "holding environment" to provide a secure-enough basis for the work, and enough leeway for temporary time out, if need be, to permit the therapy to continue without becoming chaotic. In addition to the necessity for income, food, and shelter, there must be back-up child care, if called for, and the latitude for taking leave from the job.

Of course, if the patient's functioning is sufficiently marginal, that in itself becomes the problem, and perhaps the focus of treatment must be directed toward counselling or advocacy addressing that issue. The patient's motivation should be taken into consideration in conjunction with the basic means for survival. Even a substantially practical base can be of little consequence if the patient is unwilling to tolerate the basic pain and emotional "risk" involved in therapy. The patient's motivation may also be compromised when the "support" system consists of a destructively enmeshed, even abusive family system.

It is axiomatic that, the more stable the circumstances surrounding the treatment, the more stable the treatment.

- **Step 2: Containment**

This concern may absorb a major part of the therapy. Both character work and trauma work must initially aim for containment of maladaptive, disruptive, or destructive impulses and behaviors, while the treatment also must strive to keep the trauma work contained within the character work.

Character work is focused on halting the use of maladaptive, externalized defenses where the need is for thoughtful, reasonable action. If the patient responds to the pressures of life by denying, passing the blame, or drinking or drugging excessively (for instance), the therapy needs to help the person become aware of this response, recognize its negative consequences, and begin to curtail it. This is hard work, because of the temporary satisfaction gained by these defenses.

Their interruption also cues the feelings of depression and anxiety described by Masterson (the "triad") because these defenses are supported by a belief system that associates them with approval, even survival.

This work with the maladaptive defenses could be described as the first phase of ego work with patients (the second phase concerns itself with the establishing of positive defenses). Although this phase must be substantially in place for the therapy to proceed, the therapist should be prepared for the patient's regression to this phase, especially if new levels of memory and emotion are evoked by the therapy.

Trauma work: It is generally accepted that work with trauma begins by establishing, as much as possible, a sense of safety. This may be done cognitively, by pointing out that the patient has always had a special capacity for putting away disturbing thoughts and feelings (dissociation), and that the patient can learn to use this capacity consciously and constructively. Relaxation using calming imagery is often used, and, if the therapist is a qualified clinical hypnotist, the "building" of a "safe place" in the patient's inner world is recommended. An additional hypnotic suggestion I use consists of taking things out and putting them away again (in whatever container suits the patient's own imagery); this reinforces the patient's capacity for closing up painful material as much as opening it up, and may prepare the way for later "fractionating" of abreactions (experiencing traumatic material in partial form over a series of sessions).

Interventions directed toward containing traumatic experience are important for keeping trauma work contained within the character work. To contain early treatment especially, surfacing of new insight and old traumatic experience should be minimized, as the patient will tend to manage these with maladaptive, treatment-destructive defenses. The treatment should avoid the encouragement of memories and deep feelings until the patient's adaptive defenses have been strengthened.

• **Step 3: Strengthening**

Each new step in this process overlaps with what has gone before, and gradually becomes predominant. Even as the therapy stresses functioning and containment, it must also begin to introduce healthy means of coping with what is stressful. Adaptive management of impulse, feeling, and behavior, which is a primary goal of therapy, can only begin when maladaptive ways are recognised and curtailed, and maladaptive ways can only be modified as alternatives are introduced. It probably would not be an overstatement to say that, to some extent, all elements of therapy have some place at all stages of therapy, as well.

Strengthening, therefore, is first focused on as an initiating phase of treatment, and continues to be of primary importance until negative defenses have been stopped or significantly modified, and expression of traumatic experience is under a degree of cognitive control. The stage of strengthening is one in which the aware self starts to awake, taking responsibility and eventual command of the situation. However, since therapy is often two steps forward and one step backward, strengthening is an issue that will have to be returned to regularly throughout the course of the treatment.

Character work: The strengthening phase of therapy is marked by a continual coming into consciousness of the problems of self-management. Personality disorder is partially defined by an obliviousness to self-destructive behavior and its consequences.

The initial containing phase of ego work constitutes a struggle to overcome the lure of secondary gains, habituation, and the sense that institution of new ways of behaving seems artificial. There is a sense of deprivation that must be countered, the "triadic" regression to old defenses to be met, and the belief that healthy gratification is too little, to late, and even punitive must be overcome.

But, with application and time, the balance shifts. There is a relief that comes with giving up behavior that evokes a "morning after" sense of ineffectuality.

Acting out brings disapproval and guilt. Avoidance and denial lead to disconnectedness and loss. Projection, devaluation and distancing occasion dissatisfaction and isolation. Idealization and clinging carry disillusion in their wake. The continuity of therapy acts as an "auxiliary ego" (Spitz, 1965) to help the patient "remember the morning after" at the moment of impulse. Once this learning begins to take hold, the patient starts to appreciate adaptive behavior, and the phase of strengthening comes into focus.

To continue in ego language, two important things happen in this phase of therapy. First, the executive function of the ego learns to flag problematic behavior and delay impulsive response. Second, the defensive ego practices substituting healthier, more mature behavior for destructive past activity. The ego is able to cognitively understand this process, and maintain it as steadily as possible until it leads to a new sense of well being, and begins to become self-satisfying and self-sustaining. In the case of personality disorder, it should be emphasized that this is not a steadily advancing process. There are steps backward that transiently block a sense of progress as the overall progress moves incrementally forward. The "disorders of the self triad" may appear at this stage (individuation leads to depression and anxiety, which lead to regression to old defenses), requiring renewed emphasis on containment. Here, the patient can be strengthened by a cognitive awareness that setbacks are a part of the process of psychic growth, and should be acknowledged and dealt with as an inevitable aspect of the work.

It should be noted that interventions throughout this-and the preceding-phase are primarily addressed to the ego (the function of the self that perceives and mediates the needs and requirements of psychic and social reality). These interventions support constructive ways of thinking and behaving, while discouraging those modes that impede healthy progress. Insight that evokes memory and feeling (such as emphasis on past family relationships) is to be underplayed, except for the gathering of a coherent history, and identifying superficial repetitive life patterns.

Specific ego-oriented interventions, such as confrontation, mirroring interpretation of narcissistic vulnerability, and here-and-now interpretations of the schizoid dilemma, will be discussed in the following chapters.

Trauma work: During this phase, while the patient's character is still an insecure and changeable container for intense feeling, it is wise to keep the opening up of traumatic experience to a minimum. However, as the personality strengthens, there may be a tendency for traumatic material to emerge and require constructive intervention.

If relaxation techniques are used, they should be reinforced (sometimes it is useful for the therapist to make a tape for the patient to play in between sessions). If hypnosis is used, the "safe place" and the capacity to put away that which has been taken out should be reinforced; positive memories and self-affirming attitudes should be evoked as counterbalance. Primarily, the patient should continue to use intellectual defenses to cognitively review material in a way that makes inroads on negative self-labeling (i.e.: "People who have been mistreated often think of themselves as bad, but the reality is that they have been treated badly").

The patient may be talking about traumatic happenings to an empathic listener (or anyone) for the first time. As the patient shares this information, unquestioned perceptions and beliefs about what has happened may be perceived in a more healthy light and begin to shift. Acknowledging intellectually that trauma is accompanied by feelings of fear, anger, helplessness, and guilt normalizes these feelings and strengthens the patient to handle their emergence.

The patient is also reassured, at least in a common-sense way, that certain beliefs (i.e.: those that blame the self unreasonably, or protect an aggressor) are based on a distortion.

If traumatic material does break through at this stage, it is important that the therapist also lend his or her own strength and capacity for containment. The therapist needs to hold steady during the patient's intensification of feeling, or even abreaction.

The therapist shows empathic receptivity during this turn of events by not pulling away from content and feeling, but by allowing the patient to verbalize or experience the stressful event that is coming into increased awareness. On the whole, the therapist will say little more than: "That's O.K.," "What happened next?" and "It will help if you talk, but it is not necessary to say more than you feel safe in saying at this time."

If an abreaction occurs, it is important that the patient is not considered to be having a psychotic break, but is allowing an as-yet consciously incompleted traumatic experience to complete itself in present time. The patient must be assured that the consult room is basically perceived to be in present time, and that the. therapist's voice should be considered a link to present time, while the therapist simultaneously verifies that the patient finds him or herself in a past situation (that feels like the present) that is trying to express itself, and needs to put that experience as much into words as possible. The patient should be encouraged to substitute verbal description for moving around the room. The therapist should not touch the patient during the abreaction, as the touch could be misunderstood as a part of the emerging scenario. Before the end of the session, it is important that the patient be exclusively in the same present time as the therapist, and consciously review as much as possible of the abreaction. Of course, it is necessary to be certain that the patient is sufficiently oriented to leave the session safely. Sometimes the patient may rest awhile in the waiting-room, or a nearby coffee shop, before resuming the business of the day.

• Strengthening, balance

The need to maintain evenness in the therapy is a primary responsibility of the therapist during this phase (in time, the patient will increasingly assume this task).

As the patient vacillates between modes of defense, and edges toward a deepening of feeling, the patient is moving into new psychic territory and becomes more vulnerable. The therapist needs to act as a responsible "auxiliary ego" to help guide and stabilize the patient.

As far as character work is concerned, the therapist must help the patient understand feeling rather than evoke it (i.e.: "It would not be surprising for you to feel anger," rather than "You must really feel angry about that; why don't you talk about it?"). The patient's goals at this stage are self-observation, awareness, and constructive self-direction, including the capacity to realize that moving forward tends to cause a paradoxical recoil to old defenses, and to be prepared for this.

The character work should find a balance between the realization of new perspectives (I'm beginning to like myself") and old vulnerabilities ("It frightens me to like myself"). As a rule of thumb, insight into the here and now ("I can stand up to people because I know the present is not the past") should predominate over deep insight into the past ("Now I hate my father for beating me every night"). The level of insight achieved by the progress of therapy is balanced against the capacity of newly-acquired defenses to tolerate the degree of feeling called forth.

The trauma work, in turn, needs to maintain equilibrium between the opening up of traumatic material and the increasing capacity to understand content and manage feeling. Equally important, there must be a balance between the character work and the trauma work that insures that the former predominates as the primary container of the process. The self is structured in the formation of character/personality, which shapes the self's capacity to define and operationalize its being. Unless it can be expressed through character, the potential self is dormant, and cannot negotiate the management of the outer and inner worlds.

It is a common countertransference problem for the treatment to be out of balance. Therapists have their own strengths and preferences which influence the therapy. The tendency to avoid trauma work and deal mostly, even exclusively, with character has been so pervasive in the field that it could be described as a trend. At the other extreme, trauma work may be done to the exclusion of character work, maintaining the cathartic notion that experience and memory can be expelled from the self. Realistically, whatever is opened up into consciousness becomes a part of self awareness, with perceptions and feelings to be managed and placed appropriately in perspective. The self cannot evolve into healthy consciousness if a part of it is suppressed (absence of trauma work), or is encouraged to flood other parts (lack of character work).

- **Strengthening, pacing**

There is often a tendency in the therapist to rush the patient to revelation-either of insightful or traumatic material. Conversely, the therapist may prefer to linger in a "hand-holding" mode, avoiding the impact of more assertive work. Of course, there may be a parallel tendency in the patient (especially to press for "progress," only to recoil at the difficulty of opening up).

Since the therapist acts as "auxiliary ego" in this therapeutic phase, the pacing of the therapy is largely under his or her guidance. Essentially, this consists in keeping the character work and the trauma work in balanced tandem, allowing time for one to keep pace with the other: neither can be neglected, and both should be in the therapist's awareness, whichever is being emphasized at the moment. Above all, the therapist should help the patient to continue to develop and use containment skills that allow for recuperation from and consolidation of intensive passages in the therapeutic process. These periods of consolidation should be mutually agreed upon, and should become part of the patient's awareness and practice.

• **Step 4: Cognitive and behavioral change** is the goal of short and shorter-term therapy. It is frequently defined by the point at which the patient decides to terminate treatment, and the therapist is willing to concur with the decision.

Essentially, strengthening and containment have been solidly established on a basis of sufficient functioning. That is, the patient has developed a capacity for self-observant, considered behavior, guided by a sound intellectual grasp of past history and its repetitive patterns, present responsibilities and vulnerabilities, and future goals. The patient has achieved a reasonable facility for both healthy independence and interdependence. Intellectual defenses, and the ability to take an objective view have largely replaced primitive, impulsive defenses and trauma-driven behavior.

Although some degree of deep insight and feeling has entered into this phase (all phases resonate with each other to some extent), this is primarily a stage of modification in comprehension, behavior, and life skills. Separation anxiety and abandonment depression have not been resolved, but their sporadic emergence has been prepared for. The patient now realizes that individuated, successful moments in life may occasion unexpected anxiety or sadness, and understands this is a phenomenon arising from past experience, and is transient if not acted upon. Similarly, when a traumatic reaction is cued, the patient knows this is the emergence of past experience that is factually over, although it still intrudes into the psyche in present time. With the cognitive assurance that the danger is historically past, that patient may also use acquired skills, such as relaxation exercises, to manage a disturbing episode.

This stage of treatment should be continued until it is clear that a stable-enough condition has been achieved. The situation should be discussed openly between patient and therapist, with the patient clearly assuming responsibility for understanding and control. Awareness, modified behavior, and self-directedness mark this level of treatment.

Since the emphasis has been placed on consciously-structured response and changed behavior rather than on fundamental change, the door should be left open for occasional return visits to therapy. The patient should know that there is nothing out of the ordinary about touching base for restabilization, and for management of any newly-emerging material.

It might also be noted that, because continuing therapy past this point begins to open a well of memory and feeling (and often strong transference reactions), the patient's resistance predictably rises here. Instead of seeing this resistance as a stuck point, shorter-term therapy can use it to assist closure of the process.

- **Step 5: Insight and dynamic change**

Inner change as well as outer adjustment is the goal of long-term therapy. It is here that memories and deep feelings originating in childhood have their due, and systematic abreaction of past experience may be required. Because of the intensity of this level of treatment, cognitive and behavioral change should be well in place. Following the steps of functioning, containment, and strengthening, the gains of ego-oriented shorter-term therapy provide a necessary bulwark against the stresses of working through.

Insight in long-term dynamic psychotherapy is gained through interpretation of the past roots of present symptoms and patterns. Its goal is the restructuring of the self through anamnesis-an emotional, conscious understanding of the relationships, events, fantasies, wishes, and fears that have shaped the patient's life from early times. To gain this integration of self, the patient constructs a coherent life story, as free from emotional distortion as possible that allows the patient a sense of wholeness and meaning, and frees him or her from the defensive misconceptions and repetitions that defined previous pathology.

The maturation of internalized object relations modifies the distortion of interpersonal relationships as the nature of the transference changes. As the patient comes to perceive more realistically, the self, the other, and interrelationships are comprehended in a more complex, ambivalent way. In the transference, the therapist is no longer seen as all good or all bad, nor is the relationship perceived as a repetition of the dysfunctional past relationship with the caregiver of the formative years.

The patient has learned to be discriminating, and so recognizes the remaining distortions of the nature of self, other, and relationship in contrast with a more mature, objectively-oriented view. This new capacity to distinguish reality from what is projected onto it is critical to identifying and ameliorating intrusions of past relationships and patterns into present time.

To acknowledge things as they were (and so to liberate them as they are), the patient must also face the characterological challenge of abandonment depression and separation anxiety. Trauma work now directly addresses avoided or incomplete memories to reclaim, as much as possible, the "lost" regions of the self. The feelings evoked by this process are profound, and the shift in the patient's perspective-especially regarding significant others-may be disorienting. The price for the acquisition of an integrated self is the loss of the self-and perhaps others-that one thought one knew.

Beyond the struggles to attain a coherent story, past the pain of anxiety, depression, and revelation, lies the grief that finally allows the release of old ties, and acceptance of a new state of being.

Finally, the balancing, pacing, and repeated consolidation of the therapy continues throughout long-term therapy. Under the stress of heightened feeling, the patient may regress to old, maladaptive defenses, and ego-oriented interventions may have to be reinstated for awhile, counterpoised against temporarily-suspended deep interpretation. If trauma work extends to this level, it should not outpace the limitations of character strength. And always, the patient must procede at an individual pace that permits consolidation of the work, and opportunity for restoring the self from the pressures of the process.

CHAPTER 3

CLINICAL ILLUSTRATIONS

3.1. Case Example: A Patient with Borderline Personality Disorder, Recent PTSD, and Developmental Trauma

Borderline Personality Disorder is descriptively defined by *DSM-IV* (1994) as manifesting "a pattern of instability in interpersonal relationships, self-image, and affects, and marked impulsivity" (p. 629). I will also be drawing from the dynamic formulation put forward by James F. Masterson M.D., which shows distinctive transference acting out, transferential, defensive, and object-related qualities which, in combination, are unique to borderline personality disorder (1976, 1981).

Masterson sees all personality disorder as arising from ingrained qualities established in the early developmental years of life-especially from one to three years of age. Biology and environment no doubt play their part, but it is the misattunement of the mother-child interaction that primarily sets the personality pattern. In the case of the borderline, the child's personal initiative is discouraged, while compliance with the mother's emotional state and wishes is rewarded (this may occur without conscious intention, but is pronounced and consistent enough in effect to create a pattern of response). This sets up a compliant, or rebellious, or compliant-rebellious attitude toward others, demonstrated by the growing child in all subsequent significant relationships. Needless to say, this attitude is repeated in the relationship with the therapist, first as transference acting out, then as transference, where it serves as a diagnostic tool.

Fixed, maladaptive defenses of the ego support the borderline's attitude and confuse the borderline's life. The definitive cluster named by Masterson includes:

Acting out:	behavior substituted for thought, feeling, and memory
Splitting:	the tendency to divide people and relationships into exclusively good or bad categories
Projective identification:	the (uncanny) capacity to reposition problematic emotional states into someone else's feelings
Projection:	the conviction that one's own undesireable emotional states belong to someone else
Denial:	refusal to admit the existence of a state of mind, emotion, or even facts
Avoidance:	"stepping around" a state of mind, emotion, or facts that cannot be successfully denied
Clinging:	the prototypical borderline interactive state—unquestioned attachment to a person, thing, or idea in order to minimize painful realities.

The borderline patient's internalized object relations are distinctive. Developmentally, the borderline has reached a stage where both good and bad feelings can be tolerated, but not mixed: the self, the other, and the relationship must be either good or bad (that is: if the self is perceived as good, the other is perceived as good; if the self is seen as bad, the other is seen as bad). Attempts to resolve the dilemma tend to lead to an alternation of the two, which is reflected in impulsive acting out, first one way, and then the other.

Masterson refers to these two *relational* states as the Rewarding Unit (all is approved-of, compliant, and good-feeling), and the Withdrawing Unit (all is disapproved-of, antagonistic, distanced, or in a clash). Technically, these should be referred to as "part-object relations units;" that is, each is a divided half of the mature, "whole-object relations unit" perception of individuals.

Confrontation: This is the often-misunderstood name given to Masterson's primary intervention for the borderline. Like all interventions useful for working with personality disorder, confrontation is addressed to the ego: first, to bring a maladaptive defense to conscious attention; second, to suggest the inherent self-contradiction of the defense.

The borderline sees the world in enduring maladaptive patterns that are founded on a split in attitude and belief which is supported by specific defenses. Confrontation "confronts" the defenses that maintain this split, juxtaposing what is said with what is being defended against.

By facing the patient's defensive, partial version of reality with the undivided view of the situation, the therapist momentarily helps the patient to synthesize a whole, undistorted concept of what is going on. In time, the patient integrates the process increasingly.

3.1.1. Some examples of confrontation

Acting out:	"You say you are eager to be here, yet you arrive twenty minutes late."
Projective identification:	"You tell me you are relieved to have lost your job, yet somehow I feel the atmosphere in the room is sad."
Projection:	"You assert your wife is spoiling your marriage with her moods, but you also say you are coming home late at night with no explanation."
Denial:	"How is it you claim to be mystified by your recurrent illnesses when you tell me you have been partying every night, getting no sleep, and forgetting to eat?"
Avoidance:	"How do you reconcile your statement that everything is fine with your brother when you come in with the black eye he gave you?"
Clinging:	"Do you ever wonder how come you think of your boyfriend as always caring, when you say he forgot your birthday, took your car without asking, and lost the keys without replacing them?"

3.1.2. Case Illustration

At the time she began her therapy, Sandra X was a thirty-two year old, single woman living alone. She was concerned with her difficulty in leaving her apartment (and therefore returning to her job), trouble with sleeping, and preoccupation with a hold-up that had victimized her.

She was a graphic artist, and appeared to take pleasure in presenting a creative appearance—accenting a stark outfit with dramatic or whimsical pieces of jewelry.

A handsome, slightly heavy woman, initially she wore no makeup other than black eyeliner to accentuate large, violet eyes, and fastened her long hair straight back. Looking at her, one sensed a pull between her wish to severely downplay her appearance, and to embellish it.

She was intelligent, quick and often argumentative. Through a substantial part of her psychotherapy, she frequently became self-defeated and tearful. A series of unhappy love affairs filled her adult years. Despite her clinging to her lovers, they slipped away or wrenched themselves loose from her. She was unable to recognize the negative role played by her clinging, or her choice of self-centered lovers. Instead, she dwelt upon the good times lost, and reinforced her denial by drinking too much wine and sometimes smoking pot.

Her parents were still living, and she spent many of her weekends at their home, despite a somewhat strained relationship. Her father was a retired businessman and alcoholic who passed much of his empty time delivering lectures on politics to a disinterested family. The mother was anxious and controlling-more occupied with worrying over her family than encouraging them to be concerned for themselves. There were two older brothers-one married and living far cross the country; the other still home and devoted to his computer.

Ms. X's presenting problem in therapy was a traumatic event that had threatened her vocation and her life. She had been robbed at knife-point, threatened, pushed to the ground, and her wrist broken. She had been forced to take leave from work. Since she had been accosted outside her apartment, she feared to return there, and moved in with her parents and brother.

The goals for her therapy were to return to work and to move into a new apartment. As long as her wrist was healing, the therapy seemed fairly effective-it focused on the level of present and future functioning. This was expedited by acknowledging the patient's need to talk about the assault, and to plan for her apartment-hunting and return to work.

Ms. X had demonstrated her practical competence by arranging for a leave of absence, breaking her lease and storing her belongings, and intellectually preparing to work and live independently again. However, as the wrist healed, and the time drew near to put her plans into action, resistances began to appear that indicated irresolution in both the areas of character and trauma.

As Ms. X began to plan to return to work and leave her parents' home, she experienced anxiety attacks associated with any form of transitional activity. Although her wrist was strong enough for driving the family car, she panicked at the thought of taking the wheel. She could not tolerate the sight of newspapers with their advertisements for apartments. Medication produced no effect on these attacks.

Containment was becoming the issue, if she were to initiate some forward movement. First, we established that she needed to take no action until we explored the cause of her panic.

Patient (Pt):   I can't go out there and do it all at once. I can't be on my own, afraid to come through my own front door.

Therapist (Th):   So put it in smaller pieces and see if any of
                   them are manageable.

She felt she could return to work if she maintained the
safe base of her parents' home. The anxiety attacks modified,
mainly stirred up by the transportation from home and
back. As she became accustomed to the commute, focusing
on the anchor point of her parents' home, she grew calmer
still.

It seemed that her traumatic reaction was being managed
by a little cognitive work and some desensitization.

Hopes for a return to her previous level of functioning
were soon discouraged.

After a period of successful commuting, Ms. X began to
think of moving into her next phase: reacquiring her own
apartment. The anxiety attacks began again.

This time, partializing the process was as useless as the
medication. Ms. X was terrified to relocate on her own. We
reviewed the elements that could make the situation less
evocative of her traumatic assault.

She could move to a well-lit area with a bus stop close
at hand and a doorman at the building entrance. Then she
said: "It's too hard. I couldn't have left home the first time
except for Tom. Now there's no one there."

Tom? It turned out that Ms. X had lived with her
parents until she was twenty-five. She had then moved
out to be with a boyfriend who eventually left her in their
apartment. Since then, she had been filling in his absence
with a series of lovers.

She had never left home ("individuated") on her own!

Th: Are you aware you've never set out independently
     before?

Pt: I've lived in my own place for seven years, now!

Th: Not exactly. You've maintained your own place, but you've always had a companion there.

Pt: So what? I've always paid my own rent.

Th: So the problem is, now that you have to pay your own rent, but without a companion, you discover it frightens you [confrontation of denial].

When Ms. X reacted by finding a new boyfriend and moving in with him, it became clear that the primary resistance at that time was characterological, not traumatic.

Ms. X demonstrated the acute separation anxiety typical of personality disorder: she could not part from her parents without the emotional "support" of a parent substitute. She relied on a number of defenses typical of the borderline: interpersonal clinging; acting out (including a tendency to regulate her feelings with boyfriends, alcohol, and drugs); avoidance; and denial.

Another borderline feature was her difficulty in perceiving her current boyfriend as anything other than kind and well-meaning [splitting]. He left the household chores to her, often forgot to pay his half of the rent, and refused to discuss any of this.

Th: Do you notice you describe him as loving and sharing, but describe his actions as self-serving and uncooperative?

Pt: I don't expect him to be perfect.

She held my confrontations at bay even when he began to stay out late and avoided sexual intimacy.

Th: You say he's a devoted lover, but you describe him as acting more like a roommate.

Pt: He just works late and gets tired. Why do you always pick on him?

Th: How come you see it as my picking on him when you keep bringing up reasons to question him yourself?

Pt: Well, sometimes I do worry a little about him [partial integration of confrontation], but. I know in his heart he's true to me [return to denial and the Rewarding Unit].

Persistent confrontation was strengthened by reality testing, as she noticed he was receiving frequent calls from the same woman, and was not at his office working late when she tried to reach him.

Th: Doesn't it astonish you to see how you always find a reason for his increasing detachment from you?

Pt: I just can't believe he's seeing someone else.

Th: The facts lead you in one direction, but your wishes don't want to go there.

Pt: [Starting to falter] I'm so mixed up. How can he be seeing someone else when he knows how much I need him? He says he loves me.

Th: [Gently] But his words go one way and his actions another.

Pt: [Integrating the confrontations and facing her underlying depression] I just can't live without him. I just can't face the loneliness.

Soon after, the boyfriend told her he had found the love of his life and, regretfully, she would have to find her own place. Shocked and furious, she then regarded him with hatred [shifting defensively to the Withdrawing Unit]. The anger carried her past her fears to a new apartment with a doorman on a well-lit street near a bus stop.

For a time, it seemed she had made an unexpectedly successful transition. However, her defensive spite soon ran out. She turned up at her session slurring her words and smelling of alcohol. She was trying to mask her feelings with wine and, in the evenings, marijuana.

Pt: How can I stand the loneliness when the apartment is so empty and I can't call him any more?

Th: There are other ways to fill your life besides with wine and smoking.

Pt: But I feel too paralyzed to try. Every time I try to face meeting people I just want to curl up in a ball. It's all I can do to force myself to go to work and back.

Th: So your feelings are discouraging, but you still know for a fact you can come and go at will.

Pt: I know it's how I feel, not what I can do. And I know part of this is an old problem. But don't you see-it's as if my fears became real. Whenever I go out, I see the knife again, and hear his voice-and then I remember hitting the ground . . .

The patient was hunched and beginning to shake. It was clear that her state had shifted. For the moment, she herself was confronting her characterological dilemma, and was experiencing an upsurge of traumatic recollections. It was necessary to shift the therapeutic approach to match her present state.

Th: Well, I think you're being honest with yourself to see that you are struggling with old fears of being on your own. That's the first step to overcoming those fears. But you've been severely set back by this frightening experience that even seems to confirm the old anxieties.

Pt: I thought I was getting more independent, and I just feel thrown to the ground for my insolence. I hear him over and over, saying "give me that bag" [crying] and then I feel myself falling, feel the impact, but I don't remember the pain. I'm numb. [She continues to cry without interruption.] I feel so weak and ashamed.

Th: That's what's so unfair. People who have been overpowered and hurt by a stronger person often suffer twice over-feeling the helplessness and pain, but also blaming themselves for allowing it. You were frightened, but you also felt humiliated because you couldn't fight back.

Acknowledgement of her insight as well as confirmation and clarification of her traumatic feelings, helped to strengthen Ms. X. The balance of interventions helped her to face her feelings of loneliness together with her frightening memories. This, in turn, released her from a degree of helplessness, both on the levels of character and trauma. She wiped away her tears and began to express a little more confidence in herself:

Pt: Despite it all, I think I like myself better for being on my own. It makes me feel more able to take care of myself.

Th: Would you say that taking more responsibility for yourself has given you a more effective picture of yourself?

Pt: Yes. I can say that part of my lingering fear of attack came because it made me feel so helpless, and I already felt like such a helpless baby.

For awhile, there was a period of consolidation, where the patient remained positively activated. She commuted, held her job, dated casually without excessive drinking, and relied on a small circle of friends—rather than her parents—for weekend diversion.

During this time, I maintained the rate of pacing set by the patient, supporting her gains, and did not probe for material that might open a deeper layer of feeling. Since the patient's character remained relatively stable, confrontation was only occasionally necessary, when she resorted to some over-drinking or pot-smoking on lonely weekends. Since she was able to speak freely of her traumatic episode to her friends as well as her therapist (her parents had been reluctant listeners), she found it intruding less into her practical life and thoughts.

It was nearly three years into treatment. Ms. X had, through confrontation, become aware of how she tried to manage her feelings through maladaptive defenses, knew the defenses, and counteracted them. She tolerated her fears and loneliness, and eased them with a growing social life, including cooking classes and entertaining friends at home. She developed interests in reading and music which helped her to appreciate times of solitude as well as social occasions. She took pride in her apartment, decorated it creatively, and found that she could enjoy it both in the company of others and alone. The traumatic episode began to fade, as it was fully expressed, acknowledged, and compensated for by neutral and good experiences.

Ms. X was coming to a resolution of her problem on an ego level. Conscious knowledge of her characterological susceptibilities led to her compensating for them. This strengthening of her character also helped her to better express and contain the traumatic episode.

Importantly, she had an awareness of the therapeutic steps she had taken, and had learned to talk to herself as her own therapist.

This is the point of ego adaptation at which the majority of therapies probably terminate. If the patient should decide to end the therapy here, a period of time should be allowed to assure that the adaptation is holding well enough. The patient should be able to autonomously face a significantly stressful situation with success. In the case of Ms. X, this test occurred when there was a break-in at the apartment next door.

Pt: I felt helpless again. I felt as if I would be attacked in my own bed at night. I started to dream about seeing the knife again, and being pushed down. But I said: "This is how you always defeat yourself." I told myself I could be resourceful. For a week I tipped the doorman to see me into my apartment, and I installed a Police lock. Now the initial shock has worn off, I feel safe and O.K. again.

Ms. X terminated her therapy, and seemed to have made a good practical adjustment. The few attacks of anxiety she experienced traveling were almost non-existent and competently managed; her job was going well, and she was developing a deepening, reciprocal relationship with Ed, her current boyfriend. Strangely, it was this relationship that brought her back to my office a year later.

She had matured. Her dark hair was styled and fell about her shoulders. Her large, violet eyes were dramatic as before, but now a touch of lipstick accentuated a full, sensuous mouth—she seemed to be allowing herself to have a mouth to express herself. There was a little more color in her dress. She had used her therapy to permit herself to come more into being, and was returning for further guidance.

Her anxiety had come back, but now was associated with her relationship with Ed. When they made love, she would sometimes be frozen with fear or go numb; when they slept together, she sometimes had nightmares.

Except for the disturbances in the relationship, her functioning was at a high level: she excelled at her work and enjoyed a growing circle of friends and activities. Her eating patterns were normal and, except for the nightmares, she slept well.

Containment was superficially sound. She was able to talk about her problems with Ed, and gain his emotional understanding. But neither of them had a practical or insightful grasp of her impasse, and this was taking its toll. They argued in frustration, and she began to drink more wine than her new social limit allowed. She had bouts of crying, and it was clear that the situation was deteriorating.

It was necessary to newly conceptualize her problem—to provide her with a cognitive hold, and to give a working plan to both patient and therapist. This would offer a new degree of containment to offset Ms. X's sense of consternation and helplessness.

First, we explored the possibility that physical closeness was cueing some unresolved piece of her assault trauma. When Ed playfully held her wrists, she had cried out; and though he had released her immediately, she had begun to shake uncontrollably until he disengaged all physical contact with her. Could this relate to the breaking of her wrist? There seemed to be no emotional echo: she no longer experienced dread over the assault, which had become an unpleasant, but fading memory.

She further investigated the content of her symptoms. When he had restrained her wrists, she had felt helpless, but she had also felt physically small. This connected somehow with her nightmares, which focused on a large and frightening shadow. The shadow was behind bars, but this offered no sense of security.

How about their love making? She was alarmed whenever his weight impeded her moving with relative freedom and initiative.

Foreplay above the waist was enjoyable, but foreplay below the waist and intercourse itself became "a marathon" as her sexual response turned numb and only reacted to prolonged stimulation. Sometimes these "marathons" lost all sense of sexual pleasure and became a kind of struggle.

I thought: This possibly has the sound of a childhood repetition. Small girl, big shadow, physical domination, and temporary resistance giving way after a "struggle." But Ms. X was not making this connection, so I limited my comments to saying: "These fragmentary fears and reactions sound as if they have their origin someplace else in your life besides the assault. Let's review your life generally and see if you can find a clue." I added: "You know, when you came here before, you needed to talk about present time, and I really don't know that much about your past life and how you grew up."

I was concerned about the issue of containment. There were possible indications of childhood trauma preceding the trauma of the assault. If this were so, my patient had no conscious recollection of it. If I interpreted prematurely, I could be leading my patient into a false scenario, or opening up frightening material too soon, or fixing her in an intellectualized stance. So I simply encouraged her to tell me about her background, to explore the possible means of misunderstanding of emotional and physical closeness.

Her mother, she said, worried a lot. The mother placed responsibility on her—for remaining a cheerful, outgoing advertisement for family solidarity—but was critical and insecure about her daughter's own enthusiasms and interests. She was uncomfortable with physical closeness, and hugged her child in a way that suggested formality and obligation. She never discussed sexuality with her, did not prepare her for menarche, but presented her with a book on the facts of life after her first menstruation.

Her father was distant and intellectualized, except for his bouts with alcohol, where he grew increasingly aggrieved and resentful of those who held positions of authority in his life, and had demanded sympathy from the captive audience in his household.

He would pull his daughter against him and ask her to say how much she loved and valued him. As the daughter complied, the mother would busy herself with household tasks.

"But you know," she said, "my mom and dad were hard workers who gave me the strength to stick to a job. Because of them, I was able to see myself through the assault."

"Doesn't it interest you that you've just talked about some difficult things about your parents, and now you're assuring me of what good people they are?" I returned to confrontation as her feelings about her parents began to evoke a defensive state.

'Why can't I talk about both?" [Avoidance.]

"You certainly can. But did you notice that the way you did it changed the subject?"

"Are you trying to get me to blame my parent?" [Denial, projection of conflict onto us.]

"No. Just to give me a full picture of your household. But did you see how you are trying to push away negative parts of that picture?"

"O.K. I suddenly just felt I didn't want to deal with it. It's true my parents have a strong work ethic, but sometimes I wish they'd drop it and show more warmth. It can get pretty cold around there." She recognized her defensiveness, integrated the confrontation, and began to examine her childhood.

She reflected: "I don't like to think about it, but I know my dad intimidated my mom. I think that was part of the reason she wanted me to be so cheerful. I remember he slapped her once—caught her off balance, and she fell. She had to have her wrist in an Ace bandage . . ."

Abruptly, she stopped, and her violet eyes opened wide.

"My fall! My wrist! It was sort of the same thing, except it happened to me, I could say it was wrong. We never talk about how rough and overbearing my father can be. Mother is always covering up. I've this bad feeling I've been looking at things the way mother wanted me to. There's a scary feeling to this. It feels like something is taking form and color and I want it to stop."

It was near the end of the session, and the issue of pacing was my concern—the patient was beginning to allow previously-defended material to come through.

"So you are on a useful track. Going over your early recollections gives you a change of perspective, which it often does for people."

She thought about increasing her sessions from once to twice a week. Adding sessions could help to contain and strengthen the therapy if she used more frequent contact not only to explore new territory, but also to adjust to it. On the other hand, I wanted to be sure she was not trying to hurry the process of insight. In response to my questions, she said she felt that she might be entering a new phase of therapy, and thought an extra visit would give her more time to let new issues develop. She also thought she would feel more secure having more frequent contact if she were to handle these new issues. Her reasoning seemed sound, and I agreed to the twice-a-week sessions.

For the next several weeks, she reflected on a childhood and adolescence dominated by her mother's anxiety, her father's demandingness, and her own need to be conciliatory to them both. They approved of her art work when it was conventionally pretty and could be displayed to family friends.

Ms. X was able to satisfy her own ambition to do sophisticated graphic work because it became associated with a few well-known magazines. Even then, it was the reputation of the magazines that pleased her parents, and not so much her art. For the first time, Ms. X began to acknowledge the degree to which her individuality and accomplishments had been minimized by her parents.

She wept a little, was sometimes angry, and essentially began to accustom herself to a more realistic view of her parental relationships.

Then she came late to a session.

"I didn't want to come here," she said, adding: "and I really did want to come here." She opened her briefcase and tugged out badly-folded sheets of art paper. "Look at this and tell me what it is!" She handed me semi-crumpled drawings that repeated the same theme: a hulking shadow behind bars.

'I can't draw it! Look at me—a professional—and I can't draw what's in my own head!' She ran her fingers through her hair, tossed her black mane about.

"Dammit! Something wants to be said!"

"Something want to be seen, then said."

"It feels blank. Numbness in my head. I used to think it was nothing. Now I know there's something there that's blocked out."

She missed the next session.

When she came in, I asked: "What happened?"

"I had such a hangover. I slept through work and through the session."

She had been on the verge of trauma work, and defense had intervened.

"So perhaps you drank to manage the feelings that started to come up last session."

"What were we talking about, anyway?" [Avoidance.]

"Do you prefer me to take responsibility for your memories?"

"O.K. I brought in the drawings. It was a bad place. Something is trying to surface with me. If I hold it at a distance, I feel curious about it. But, like last week, if I let it in close, I get really scared." [Quick integration of confrontation, showing some readiness to do trauma work.]

Assuming a more cognitive, trauma-oriented approach, I said: "You know, a memory is about something in the past. The scared feeling you get probably comes from a memory, and so it comes from the past, too. The threat is over, now-no longer in the present."

"But it feels like now. Like something terrible is going to happen to me any minute."

"Feelings always seem to be in present time—it's what makes us try to attach them to present facts even when they come from the past."

Educative information about feelings and the nature of traumatic states helps to contain and strengthen the process. In terms of trauma work, especially, some distress is modified when the therapist shows understanding and helps the patient to make sense of a baffling situation. Even in terms of character, intensity of emotion may be counterbalanced by the strengthening of intellectual defenses.

Ms. X was on the edge of moving forward, and was shifting her emotional priorities to fear of activating traumatic states that were once genuinely overwhelming. My interventions had to shift accordingly, from confrontive to supportive and educational. And I had to be prepared to shift back again, should she reinstitute maladaptive characterological defenses. Balance had become an important element in the advancement of the therapy.

She wanted to see how far back she could take her childhood memories.

"My mother always seems to have been the same-anxious and deferring to my father. My father must have been drinking 'way back, because I don't remember a time when it started. I just know I was about ten when I figured out why he acted differently on weekends, and why mother tried to keep me out of his way. Strange . . ." I waited. "It's embarrassing. Talking about my father on weekends, I get this sexual feeling. Now I realize I get that feeling with my father after I've been away and come to visit him. It doesn't feel good. It feels humiliating. I don't want to talk about it."

However, she was able to continue the next session. "That bad sexual feeling—it goes 'way' back, but I can't attach it to anything except being with my father. Do you think he did something to me? So long ago I don't have any real memory of it-just this feeling? The idea feels crazy. What do you think?"

I had to be careful to be neither leading nor rejecting. "I don't know. I know you have disturbing sexual sensations that seem to originate at a time in your life when your memories were not verbal, but were held in your feelings. You associate these feelings nowadays to your father's presence, but the reason for that is unknown. You also associate these feelings with a sense of humiliation, and it is likely you are protecting yourself from an intensification of that feeling, and that you won't allow yourself to be more specific until you feel prepared to be."

I was concerned with the pacing of the process. Although she was repelled by her thoughts, she was also animated and curious. She wanted to push toward knowledge, as many patients do before experiencing the impact of revelation. Her character defenses were still shaky, and I had no way to judge the depth and intensity of what seemed to be a traumatic experience in her past.

I told her what I tell patients who are at this juncture: "The self is wise, and apparently has protected you from knowing more than you needed to know up to now. There may or may not be much more to know, but it works best if you don't try to force things.

If you continue to hold steady, not drink, and explore the situation in words, your unconscious mind may have more to tell you."

For a few weeks she remained in a stuck place—unable to understand more, but haunted by what she felt was important knowledge just beyond her conscious awareness.

"It's so frustrating," she said, "to be closed off from my own knowledge. I feel doubly humiliated."

We talked about where she had lived in her early childhood. She clearly recalled the house she had primarily grown up in, then grew curious about an apartment the family had occupied until she was four.

"I want to remember my bedroom—I have such an intense feeling about it. It's the atmosphere-it seems to draw me there. I can't see it all clearly, maybe because it's nighttime, but the curtains are catching the streetlight and making patterns on the ceiling. The patterns are moving-maybe from the headlights of a car-I see faces and shapes in the shadows. The rest of the room is dark except for the wall beside my bed. There's enough light from outside so I can reach up and *see* the shadow of my hand."

She paused, looking puzzled. "But pieces are missing. It's not the darkness. It's as if sections of the room are blurred out, or just not there. This is frustrating.

The next session she arrived looking animated. She took an envelope from her purse. She removed a series of photographs, and began to deal them out on the desk.

"Look at this! Mother, father, and me when I was three years old! Look how tightly daddy is holding me while mom looks away, and how I'm trying to get her attention! And the other pictures are the same. Daddy always holds me, while I reach out to her, or look at her, and she won't look at either one of us."

"What do you make of it?"

"Well, dad sort of takes me over, and she goes into the distance, even when I reach for her."

"What does that mean to you?"

"It just seems to confirm something. As if she won't protect me."

"Why should she need to protect you?"

She put down another photo—a child in a crib, wide-eyed and retreating against the crib bars in the far corner.

"See how apprehensive I look! (How could my parents want to keep this photo?) And look—look at the bars and see how the camera flash throws their shadow on the wall! That's my drawing of the bars! Now I understand why the figure in the drawing isn't safe behind bars. The streetlight is casting the shadow of the figure and the shadow of the bars against the wall. He's leaning over the crib."

"You said 'he.'"

She paused. "I don't know why. I just said it. I suppose it would be my father, but I don't really know. But I have a bad feeling, and all this seems to fit together somehow. Would my own father abuse me? It feels unreal and it feels probable, all at the same time."

She left looking excited and also troubled.

I received a phone call the next day asking for an emergency appointment. She had waked up in the middle of the night, struggling and crying out.

"It was awful. Even when I was awake, I didn't know where I was for awhile."

She folded her hands, looked down at them, tried to compose herself.

"I dreamed something was closing out the light, and then my body started to prickle. I started to feel terrified and sexually aroused at the same time. I can't describe it, except that I rushed awake in terror I was going to die." She stared at me earnestly. "Where is this going? I've had nightmares before, but no waking memory of them. Did my father abuse me? My body, my feelings seem to know something I don't know. Why am I scared of Ed when we make love? Why do I go numb? Can you hypnotize me to find out?"

I acknowledged her apprehension, told her that hypnosis was a possibility, but that it seemed unnecessary. Her traumatic experience seemed to be emerging at a controlled pace, without the need for additional intervention.

She was increasingly absorbed in the riddle of her early years, and arrived soon after with an expression of intense elation.

"It was my father. My mother caught him fondling me in my crib. She says he was drunk, but knew enough not to do it again after she caught him."

This was an unusual turn of events—corroboration of abuse from someone who was afraid of the molester.

"How did she come to tell you this?"

"She didn't want to. She tried to evade me and deny anything ever happened." Ms. X sat back, seeming satisfied. "But I threatened her. I said, if she didn't tell me whatever she knew, I'd go to my father and ask him."

Once more, anger had mobilized her and carried her to a stronger position. And it was unusually fortuitous that her assertiveness had met with corroboration of the abuse. On the whole, I have found that patients who suspect they have been molested in childhood hesitate to disturb the family silence, and when they do, are frequently met with denial or anger.

She conceded: "I feel sort of badly that 1 threatened her. She's so afraid of him. It makes me feel like him to threaten her."

"So now that you refuse to act like a victim, you think you must have become an abuser?"

"I suppose it's my right to know . . . my life. There is a sickening feeling about it, though."

"Now you are more aware of the facts, the feelings you numbed at the time may get stronger-you were too young to master them then, but perhaps you will take your adult strength to master them now and complete the memory." (I was explaining the mechanism of abreaction to her to provide a conscious container for the possible emergence of further experience.)

Not long after, late at night, my answering service called me. Ms. X had awakened in the middle of a nightmare and was barely able to distinguish past from present. I returned her call.

She was distraught, but able to tell me what was happening.

"Please help me. My hands are going numb. I feel so scared. Something is crawling on me. I can't stand it. Please help me!"

I spoke as calmly and simply as I could: "It's all right. You don't feel safe, but you really are safe. This is an unfinished piece of your past that needs to express itself. Once you let it through, it will become just a memory and begin to fade. Just let it be, and tell me all about it. "I'm here."

"Please don't go away!"

"I'll stay as long as you need to feel better. Do you want to tell me about what's happening to your hands?"

"No! I want this to stop! Help me!"

I had helped patients through abreactions over the phone, and knew it could be done. In fact, abreactions may occur between sessions despite efforts at containment. The period of sleep, especially, is a vulnerable time when states of consciousness become blurred. It is also possible to close up an abreaction over the phone, and this I attempted to do, especially since she had clearly requested it.

"Listen to my voice . . . let it be your anchor to present time. I'm right here, and I will help you."

"Please, please let me go!" [Appealing to the other person in the traumatic experience.]

"How are you being held?"

"My wrists!"

"Are you holding the phone?"

"Yes."

"So you are able to move your hands after all, and you can move them more to help yourself more. Is there a light on?" "No." "Is there a light nearby?" "Yes, on the bedside table." "You can reach for that light and turn it on." "I can't move." "But see, you already dialed the phone. You are talking to me because you called me in present time, and the past is growing dimmer as I speak. Your hands can feel, and you can begin to feel your way to the light-switch. Follow the sound of my voice in present time, and turn on the light now."

This exchange continued for awhile until she turned on the bedside light. She continued to be disoriented awhile, and I persisted in a reassuring tone of voice, encouraging her return to present time.

Finally: "I'm O.K. now, just shaky. What was it?"

"Sounded like unfinished business from the past intruding into the present."

"Somebody held my wrists and was touching me. It's so clear I can almost see it."

"Let that go for now, and let it fade into the background. We can discuss it in your session tomorrow. How are you now?"

"Something feels like letting go. I can hang up, now. "I'll get some milk and read awhile."

"Fine. Just remember how you helped yourself, and how I'm here to help you."

Abreactions are often at the center of trauma work, and must be handled in their own way. The therapist should acknowledge that the emerging past experience is unintegrated, and therefore is felt to be still active in present time when the evolving memory is bought closer to the surface by some triggering event. This is an experience that has been locked in discrete states to prevent the psyche from being flooded. In therapy, as the self grows stronger, and can manage previously-overwhelming material, these states are activated and synthesized, the perception of the experience is completed, and becomes a full memory with the capacity to fade in time. This process, if forced or cut off abruptly, may retraumatize the patient by evoking too much to deal with, without some form of resolution. In this instance, I helped Ms. X to gain some increased knowledge and mastery of her symptoms, which allowed her to voluntarily put them away pending further work [to fractionate the abreaction].

The therapy facilitated this process, as I encouraged Ms. X not only to experience her trauma emotionally, but also reassured her that she was "living" the past in present time.

The oscillation of traumatic experience with anchoring in the present helped her to titrate the process.

She spent the next few sessions consolidating the impact of this happening.

"So my nightmares have been my attempt to bring my past into the present so I can resolve it." She had grasped the distinction between traumatic dreams and conventional dreaming.

And then: "But how could my father do this to me? It wasn't only the touching—he terrified me! How could I live with him all these years? How could I listen to his political drunken crap and stay in the same room with him? No wonder it makes me feel weird on weekends: on weekends he's drunk, and he was drunk when he molested me!" She added: "And how can I let myself drink? I drink to get away, and it just gets me closer to him."

Gradually, the stronger she felt in the situation (familiarity helped, and anger), the more she began to experience uncomfortable, sensations: fear, humiliation, and genital arousal. She continued to function relatively well, maintaining her job and her relationship with Ed. But, again, work and love were increasingly impaired by her tension, shortness of temper, disturbed sleep, and trouble tolerating sexual closeness . . .

She arrived in a state of frustration beyond tears. "I can't stand this! I know what I know, but it feels as if it's behind a thin wall, and I can't get through. Myself, my own experience, is on the other side of that wall, and I am walled off from me. My body feels it, my feelings feel it, sometimes I can even see flickers of it, but I have no sense of really getting it. It isn't the way it was with the assault. I've been through that I remember going through that, and it's over. I keep telling myself my mother saw it—it happened the way

I feel it happened. So why can't it be clear in my mind? Why can't I remember?"

"Please," she asked, "can't we try hypnosis?"

I will occasionally use hypnosis as an adjunct to long-term psychotherapy, So I gave her request careful consideration. A major criterion must be that the patient's character work has been significantly accomplished. Hypnosis, like deep interpretation, can stir up disturbing memories and feelings that must be managed by adaptive defenses, along with the capacity to delay impulse, reflect, and integrate material that may change basic perspective on one's life. For this reason, I had refused Ms. X's initial request for hypnosis. At the time, she was "managing" feelings with denial, avoidance, and acting out, and I did not wish to provoke more of this by uncovering new stressors. Her first request seemed based on a "magical" concept of "cure."

Now, however, Ms. X's defenses were much more adaptive, and her resistance seemed mostly trauma based: part of her still feared the formation of complete, conscious memory. Tolerating this change might be no worse than struggling with the stuck place she found herself in, with her life compromised by half-evolved traumatic experience. Would it be appropriate to *not* use an established intervention, in which I was trained, where conventional psychotherapy seemed to have reached a limit?

Furthermore, it was my experience that solid character work laid the basis for the emergence of traumatic experience. The experience either would appear spontaneously (sometimes unexpectedly), or require a minimum of hypnotic intervention to come through.

In addition, the traumatic experience Ms. X sought to consciously complete had been corroborated by her mother. The problem was not one of establishing facts, but of integrating states of awareness.

I agreed, therefore, to offer Ms. X a series of hypnotic sessions.

I introduced hypnosis to her as a state of relaxation in which she could exercise her own skills in shifting into or out of any state of mind she chose. I assured her of her mind's capacity to go to and return from wherever it would, and to use my voice as a guide back to the room in present time. I helped her to use pleasant recollections and imagination to create a place of peacefulness and safety in her mind that would be her unique haven. She also knew that, if she raised her left hand, palm up, my voice would lead her back to the office and conscious wakefulness.

She spent a few sessions learning to be as relaxed and comfortable as possible with this situation. Especially, she grew familiar with her safe place-the bank of a mountain stream. The stream was brilliant with shining ripples and bright pebbles, and was watched over by friendly animals.

On the fourth session, I invited her to enter a completely clear space in her mind, and there—if she chose-to reconstruct her bedroom of three-years-old. She tried to do so, then said the space was unclear and filled with bad feelings. She decided to return to an unaltered state. Although this was disappointing for her, it advanced her ability to delimit, or "fractionate" her hypnotic experience. This self-protective skill is important for maintaining the patient's tolerance for the work. The hypnotic experience may begin slowly, but once started, may move along with rapidity and increasing intensity. Dividing the work into segments is a way to titrate the process. Incidentally, it also makes the work more adaptable to the length of the office visit.

The next session, she allowed herself to see the shadow of the crib bars, then the shadow of the figure. As she focused her attention on the figure itself, she began to grow restless and frightened, and asked to return to the room.

The next session, she shook as she felt her hands being restrained, and the session after, shifted in pain as she felt fingers intruding into her vagina.

She sat facing me during these sessions. Afterwards, I would spend some time with her to ask what she recalled of the session, to give her time to begin to consolidate new information, and to become re-oriented in present time. I asked her to focus her vision on the near, middle, then far distance, and assured myself she was out of the altered state before closing the session.

During the last several sessions, she became aware that she was recalling more than one happening. She reported she could perceive her father clearly, now, and that he wore different clothing during different episodes. He was rougher at times, squeezing her body, and slapping her if she started to whimper. These sessions were among the most difficult, because of the intensity of her fear during the abreaction, and because of her disgust afterward, when she concluded that the abuse had been more extensive than she had realized, and that her mother might have been aware of it.

The abreactions stopped after that. Perhaps her mother had interceded, after all, or perhaps the move from the apartment to her parents' present home had changed things. In their new home, her bedroom had been adjacent to the living-room, which would have afforded less privacy for secret activities.

She emerged from the series of hypnotic sessions with deeply mixed feelings. She felt whole for the first time, yet she resented the loss of her past for so long, and deplored the impact it had had upon her life. With the consolidation of memory, her nightmares steadily diminished, and physical intimacy with Ed became increasingly satisfying. She felt both liberated and betrayed.

One day, she tried to face her father. When he understood where the conversation was going, he refused to discuss any part of it, called her "a mental patient," and slammed into his study. She was able to shout after him: "You're the mental patient!" and then boycotted her parents' household.

For a period of several weeks, she was clear, satisfied, and free from symptoms. She felt she had brought the family secret into the open, and was pleased with her own courage.

We both felt the case was again reaching closure.

Then one day she came to her session looking grim, and asking for my support in taking her father into court.

"He needs to suffer more."

I explored her feelings with her, and empathized with them. However, I questioned her wish.

Would she be accomplishing anything besides losing more time and energy over her father?

Why did she choose to remain tied to her past?

How could she expect her mother to support her in court?"

As I had previously warned her, my testimony would be compromised because I had used hypnosis.

Above all, I stressed that "Law suits are not a stage of therapy. If you want to take this to court, it should be after you have finished your therapy: after you have resolved your feelings and got your life in order. Otherwise, to go to court will open up anything left to open, and tear at the strengths you are building. Going to court is not a method of termination. If you have gone beyond your fear and anger, left what happened in the past, but feel justice still needs to be done-objective justice, not personal revenge-you might want to consider litigation. If, for instance, your father was baby-sitting for neighbors' children or grandchildren, you might feel a moral need to take action.

But why take a chance at derailing your work with yourself, or even re-traumatizing yourself—either by winning or losing-for the sake of vengeance? Doesn't vengeance simply lock you into another kind of abusive relationship with your father?"

As I listened to myself, I realized I had automatically started to shift into a confrontive mode, and wondered whether I was subliminally picking up a resurgence of characterological defense.

I was not concerned with the damage she might do to her father, who was responsible for his actions, but was refusing to come to any kind of reconciliation. I was concerned with the damage she might do to herself. As I had mentioned, she could be re-traumatized even if she won, and the considerable chances of losing or suffering a countersuit could be devastating.

"It's all your fault!" Her violet eyes were dark with accusation. "You compromised me by hypnotizing me! Now my testimony won't stand up in court."

It was no use reminding her that this had been carefully discussed in advance, and that she had signed a permission slip permitting me to hypnotize her—a slip that included the warning that the use of hypnosis would legally compromise any possible litigation connected with the treatment.

"You didn't see I was too desperate to make a decision. You just let it happen."

Her attitude and accusations persisted, while I found myself feeling ineffectual and even frightened. My reactions intensified when she threatened to take me to court.

"It's a double betrayal. First him, and now you."

Something rang a bell. She was treating me like her mother, and I was feeling helpless and alarmed like her mother. Was this a regression to borderline transference acting out, and the countertransferential response it induced? She had had no difficulty assessing her anger at her father, but had backed away from feelings about her mother after her initial reaction.

She continued: "You were supposed to be there for me, but now you've pulled out. You've left me with no one."

"Do you think you could feel this way about your mother, too?"

"Yes. You've all betrayed me and left me all alone."

She hurried out in a rage, leaving me worried for the next three weeks. First she missed a session, then she was drunk when I telephoned. On the brink of resolving major emotional and life issues, she had regressed to her original borderline defensiveness. I should have been prepared for this, recalling the formula of the disorders of the self triad: "Separation—individuation leads to anxiety and depression, which lead in turn, to the reinstitution of old defenses." Successfully completing her therapy would mean that Ms. X would have to use her new confidence in herself to assert herself and live a life separate from her parents. This would involve perceiving her parents on a realistic, present-time basis, free as possible from old fears and longings. She would have to let go of the retaliatory anger that might still hold her to her father, and would have to face that her mother was a frightened and therefore limited person who was unable to defend her own child, or at the very least, prevent that child's abuse. She would have to stand on her own, as a person stronger than her own parents, accept however that affected her relationship with them, and move on into her own life.

Then at last she came in.

Yes," she said, I feel betrayed by my mother."

Her last upsurge of borderline defense had given away before the strong intellectual and creative defenses she had built, and in the light of the therapeutic alliance between us. She had been reasoning with herself, and, when words failed, had been making sketches of the different relationships between herself and her father, her mother, and me.

In the sketch with her father, they had been turned away from each other. In the sketch with her mother, the mother had been turned away from the daughter's reaching arms. In the sketch with me, we had been turned toward each other, holding hands reassuringly. She realized she had seen me negatively (split her bad feelings from her good ones about me) in order to make me the scapegoat for her remorse. She was able to shift from borderline global indictment of me, to neurotic transference, which was able to see the negative within a positive-negative mixture.

"You've worked with me for six years. You had patience with my drinking; you looked at my drawings and photos and gave me the courage to talk to my mother; you had the skill to hypnotize me and help me to be whole; I faced my father because you were there; and yes, you didn't rubber-stamp my tantrum and give me permission to get involved in some court thing with my parents. You really have been there. So why should I hate you?

"It isn't you I hate. You're right. It's mother." She faltered. "But she was all I had. Why did she let it happen? Why did she hide the truth and protect him?" Her expression became grave. "And you know, I don't think she's telling me the truth now. I'm really sure he did it to me more than once. Maybe she didn't know, or maybe she stopped him by catching him by mistake. But what did she think he was doing in my room so often when he was drunk? Was she relieved he was letting her alone? Was she afraid he'd knock her down if she tried to stop him?"

The defensive energy of her anger collapsed, leaving her drained and bitter. The abandonment depression, so long below the surface of her mood, was no longer warded off, but permeated her emotional world.

For weeks she came in and sat in silence, or spoke of a deep well of personal loss.

"I never had a father. I never had much of a mother, either. They took away my childhood, and because I couldn't remember, I messed up my adulthood myself. Why couldn't they at least confess, express regret, give me back myself? All the nightmares, the drinking, the affairs with no pleasure! Just because I kept trying to remember and couldn't! I might as well have been dead half the time. I feel like being dead, now."

Her depression, heartfelt for many weeks, begin to become repetitious. A stubbornness entered it, so that I knew it had taken on a defensive quality. She needed to let go of it all.

Finally, she recognized her own defensiveness and questioned it.

"I'm acting lost instead of just letting myself feel lost, aren't I? I keep protesting and hanging on as if it would change something. Why can't I just accept what happened, and move on?"

"It's sad," I said, "but after all these years, your parents haven't really found any comfort to offer you."

There was a silence, and then she leaned forward with her face in her hands and began to sob. She continued for many minutes, and only repeated "mother" a number of times. At the end of the session, she composed herself and said "It's over."

So transference acting out had given away to transference; anger at me had made place for anger at the mother; and resistance had at last dissolved into the central grief of a child longing for a mother's protection.

She continued to come in, mostly to grieve, for several months after that. Since then, she has returned periodically to resolve the stress of achievement (promotion at work) or threatened separation (she and Ed nearly parted in the process of learning to argue with each other).

Old scars still remain, and she works hard to solidify a sense of trust in herself and others. She and her mother have made a wary truce, since Ms. X, as a result of her grief, allowed herself to acknowledge the extent of her mother's weakness. Ms. X and her father remain estranged, and meet neither in nor out of court.

3.2. A Patient with Manifest Narcissistic Personality Disorder and Developmental Trauma

DSM-IV (1994) gives the primary diagnostic features of narcissistic personality disorder as "a pervasive pattern of grandiosity, need for admiration, and lack of empathy." The narcissist has a "grandiose sense of self-importance," and expects to be recognized as special, yet "their self-esteem is almost invariably very fragile" (p. 658).

Masterson (1981) expands this description to include two faces of pathological narcissism: manifest narcissism and "closet" narcissism. The first is similar to the DSM-IV type, while the last(featured in the next chapter) "presents him/herself as timid, shy, inhibited, and ineffective—only to reveal later in therapy the most elaborate fantasies of the grandiose self" (pp 7-8).

The narcissist, like the borderline, suffers from a developmental arrest that has its roots in the early years of life. Masterson observes that the mother-child relationship of the practicing sub-phase of separation-individuation (Mahler, 1972, pp. 123-127) has qualities that carry over into the later years in a fixed, inappropriate way.

The practicing child does not yet have a clear sense of separation from the mother, and assumes her uninterrupted protection and esteem. The mother supports this sense of oneness as she mirrors the child's confidence and anticipates the child's needs. The demands of reality and the child's evolving individuation eventually question this sense of blissful merger, and the healthy youngster begins to accept the challenge of autonomy. But when the mother consistently disregards individuative tendencies and encourages continued grandiosity and merging, the child begins to perceive separation as a negative, unloved state. A fixed, idealized connection that elevates the self and other to a mutually idealizing state may replace the realistic differentiation of healthy growth. The interruption of this condition is experienced as a fragmentation of being.

These fixed characteristics are acted out in therapy as the narcissist seeks admiration and mirroring from the therapist. If the patient feels sufficiently respected and understood, an idealized sense of self is reinforced that brings with it a sense of unity with another who is also idealized and not clearly differentiated from the self. This provides the basis for treatment, which otherwise would be considered demeaning or hostile to the patient's sense of elevated oneness.

The need of the narcissistic patient to feel understood, important, and idealized can be a stumbling-block for therapists who themselves feel demeaned when promoting this transferential state. It needs to be stressed that the narcissist cannot be met on any other ground. To perceive oneself as admired by someone who is consequently admired, is a position of safety for the narcissist—a reclaiming of a protected, unassailable world. To be questioned, interpreted, or shown any sign of difference is to be attacked. Questions and interpretations take away the sense of special oneness, and evoke a sense of fragmentation.

Of course, to acknowledge that the world is a place of differences with few harbors of total congruence is the substance of the working through. But the narcissistic patient will not entertain such a concept except from the secure (if illusory) base of an idealized relationship.

Idealization, therefore, is the primary defense of pathological narcissism, along with *devaluation* (to discount anyone who threatens the importance of the self), and *detachment* (to sever the self from anyone or thing seen as devaluing).

The defenses shared with the borderline are *acting out, splitting, projective identification, projection, denial,* and *avoidance. Idealization* rather than *clinging* is the defensive mode of attachment.

The narcissistic patient's internalized object relations are split more severely than the borderline's.

Both live in a world of severely demarked "good" and "bad." But the borderline can relate (if unhealthily) through either feeling state. The narcissist only relates to "good"—a designation of "bad" dismisses the other to outer darkness. For "bad" equals "different" and evokes a sense of fragmentation. This is why so secure a sense of oneness, or "good," must be established with a narcissist before the idea of the realistic co-existence of "bad" is even acceptable for consideration.

Mirroring Interpretation of Narcissistic Vulnerability. Narcissists experience a differing point of view as an attack. If interpretation and confrontation represent intolerable points of view, how does the therapist speak therapeutically with a narcissist? Masterson (1993, pp. 76-79) has developed a specialized form of interpretation that addresses the narcissist's vulnerability and need to defend against a threat to that vulnerability in a way that allows the patient a degree of new perspective while continuing to feel understood. The key to this intervention is the acknowledgment of the patient's pain when the sense of vulnerability is breached, and the need to protect the self from this pain. In this way, defenses may be delineated without the patient feeling attacked, for the defenses are identified as self-protective and understandable (which once was true in the patient's early life).

The formula for this intervention is "pain . . . self . . . , defense," and can be used as follows:

Grandiosity (self-idealization):	"It disappoints you not to get credit where it is due you, so you protect yourself by stressing your accomplishments. "
Devaluation:	"It is so distasteful for you to feel attacked, that you protect yourself by putting the other person in his place."

Detachment:	"What I just said doesn't show understanding, so you dismiss it by ignoring it."
Acting out:	"It offends you when I disagree with you, and you want to place yourself on firmer ground by leaving the session early."
Projective identification:	"I seem to sense disappointment in the room—I wonder if you've somehow buffered yourself from it, and I'm sensing it alone."
Projection:	"I think you feel offended by your friends' criticisms, and repay the compliment by pointing out their faults. "
Denial:	"It pains you to hear disagreement, so you deflect it by dismissing it completely."
Avoidance:	"I think I just disappointed you, because you seem to have protected yourself by I changing the topic. "

(Mirroring as the sole intervention may be necessary if the patient is feeling excessively vulnerable. Eg.: "I've disappointed you. You came here to be understood, and I've let you down." It should be noted that it is the patient's feeling that is being mirrored—facts should not be distorted. Although the patient may argue the facts of the matter, the real issue for the narcissist is feeling understood.

There is a division in the field regarding the usefulness of mirroring. Since mirroring supports regressive defense, the

Masterson approach considers it a regressive intervention. Other approaches hold that mirroring strengthens existing defense in order to ready acceptance of more adaptive defenses. I have sometimes used mirroring in this case when the patient's anxiety level seemed anti-therapeutic, but this does not exemplify the Masterson approach, which would exclusively use mirroring interpretation of narcissistic vulnerability.

3.2.1. Case Illustration

Harry H, 59 years old, was the owner of a small real estate company. The success of the company fluctuated, as did his relationship with his partner. His marriage of thirty years was also in a changeable state, and was headed for divorce. His three grown children all seemed to have acted strongly on their parents' emphasis on material acquisitions, and their father's driving ambition. The oldest, a son, pushing himself to accomplish, gained marginal success, an ulcer, and a constant need for his father's approval.

The middle child, a girl, was an aggressive achiever on her way up the corporate ladder. The youngest, a girl, reigned over a following of attentive boyfriends, while wearing only the latest fashions and running up her assortment of credit cards. Mr H presented with a sense of frustration, depression, and loss—his problem was situational and characterological, but not traumatic. The traumatic elements would emerge as his personality disorder modified.

Mr H had put on a little too much weight. His hair was greying and slightly balding above regular features that could turn contemptuous or unexpectedly boyish. Although he wore expensive clothing, he maintained a mildly disheveled look: his tie would be loosened and off center, or his shirt partly pulled out. He spoke quickly, articulately, and used hand gestures for emphasis. He wore a heavy gold ring with his initials engraved on it.

3.2.1.1. Presenting problem

Mr. H described a personal crisis that had traumatic overtones. He believed his world had fallen apart overnight. Inexplicably, he thought, his wife had declared she was "fed up," and was suing for divorce. His partner was tampering with the books and would have to be confronted. Business was failing. His son lacked push and was too dependent on him. His oldest daughter, by contrast, contacted him rarely and ignored his advice. His youngest, his little princess, was surely going to bankrupt him. To ice the cake, he was almost 60 years old, and his father had died at 61. Was his health poor? He had to be careful of his high blood pressure, but his father had keeled over entirely unexpectedly, and in apparent top physical condition.

Mr. H kept up an almost jaunty manner while presenting his situation. He seemed to want to give the impression of a man able to carry a heavy burden lightly, and with humor. He also seemed to be maneuvering me into becoming his responsive audience. I felt a double reaction—to argue or admire—noted it as probably a diagnostic clue, and settled for a neutral stance with a touch of mirroring.

3.2.1.2. History

Mr. H was the youngest of two brothers, the sons of immigrant parents. The father worked long hours establishing a dry-cleaning business—he made a college education possible for his sons, and was determined to see them become professionals. The mother worked with her husband, making clothing alterations. She supported his ambition for their sons, but also protected them from his demands and domineering temper. She favored her youngest, Harry, and made him her confidant.

Isolated by barriers of culture, class, and family ambition, Mr. H had a lonely childhood and adolescence. He had difficulty concentrating, and spent extra hours over his books. A good report card meant approval from his father and praise from his mother, while bad grades brought disgust and grief, respectively.

Unable to gain acceptance to medical school, or to succeed in passing the bar examination, he finally began to build a real estate business with the help of a wife as ambitious as his parents. His wife also provided the social life he had rarely experienced. His family grew, his business prospered, and he took on a partner.

However, his early middle years were darkened by losses. His brother suffered a mental breakdown while starting a second career at dental school, and committed suicide. His father died suddenly, probably of a stroke, and his mother passed away soon after, following a harrowing series of heart attacks.

Bereft of his family of origin, Mr. H, in his late middle years, focused all his concerns on his immediate household and real estate business. The partial collapse of this core of his reality brought him to psychotherapy.

3.2.1.3. Psychotherapy

Mr. H adjusted his chair to a more commanding spot and scrutinized me.

"You could do better than this stuff"—he indicated my furniture—"I can give you the name of a good wholesale place. Just mention my name."

"Thanks, but these things have been with me a long time."

"They look it. This is just some friendly advice. You want to impress people when they walk in."

I felt devalued by way of my furniture, and realized that my patient was assuming authority. The diagnostic signs of the manifest narcissist appear quickly. I tried to reclaim my position.

"Tell me, what brings you here?"

"No 'thank you'?" He was half-joking.

"For what?"

"For the advice, of course. Are you usually this slow on the uptake?"

I decided he had a point and began to mirror him: "Sorry. I should have appreciated your concern; thanks for the offer and for your good humor about it." [Acknowledging my "rebuff" and his attempt to joke it off.]

He settled back in his chair, apparently mollified.

"Let's get on with it, doc. I don't mind telling you this isn't usually how I spend my lunch hour."

The easy part came next, as I asked him to tell me his background. He told me his story seriously, especially becoming solemn at describing his relationship with his parents. He wiped his eyes (with the back of his hand, like a little boy) while speaking of his mother. He spoke briefly about when his brother "croaked," detaching himself quickly from the topic.

The hard part for him was addressing the complex of events that made up his presenting problem:

"Doc, how can I deserve this now, when I should be successful and happy with my family around me? I earned it; I created it; it's part of me. I worked; I gave; I deserve gratitude. My wife, my partner, my kids, they'd be nowhere without me.

"But I tell you, the worst is this feeling I've been left alone to die. I think—why are they leaving me when I have only one year to go?"

"This is painful to think about. What does your doctor say?"

"Doctors! My dad had a clean bill of health—then wham! He took my mother with him, and now I figure he's going to take me."

I decided that Mr. H's separation anxiety had focused powerfully on the idea of death, and that probably it was a defense that would have to stay intact for now to protect against his intolerable sense of loss. I would try to help him contain this anxiety by focusing on the more concrete problems of the here and now. These present issues in themselves threatened his functioning both at home and at work, and approached traumatic proportions (this was the third time the structure of his life had been threatened; once when he failed to achieve a profession; twice when his immediate family had died; and now when his entire sum of success was being demolished, leaving him with fears of death).

Since the patient was in a crisis situation, I thought I should place the therapeutic emphasis on strengthening of Mr. H's self-esteem. I planned to be an empathic listener who understood his point of view, and thus lowered his need for unrealistic and grandiose defense. He might then have better access to his healthy intellectual and assertive capacities.

3.2.1.4. Introductory phase

During the first few months of treatment, the pacing of the work went ahead carefully. It was necessary to mirror Mr. H's sense of vulnerability so that he would feel understood—and would begin to idealize me in return. The transference acting-out shifted from his need to maintain his grandiosity by putting me (or my furniture) down, to a sense of our being merged in a self-satisfied emotional entity.

Pt: I get all the lousy luck.

Th: Do you think you might play some part in this?

Pt: You trying to tell me I brought this on myself?

Th: Just trying to say you can have some control over what starts with you. You can be less helpless.

Pt: Now it's all my fault, plus I'm just a helpless wimp.

Th: Sorry. I guess that sounded like an attack. There's no question you've had more than your share of tough times.

Pt: You bet your tail. What's with you today?

Th: I didn't show understanding. You had to protect yourself by challenging me.

Pt: I thought you knew me.

Th: I disappointed you.

Pt: That's what I like about you, doc. You admit when you're off base. You keep an open mind, like me.

As time passed, it was possible to increase interpretation of defenses, as mirroring established a sense of idealized unity. We could begin to tackle his problems more directly.

Patients who enter therapy in crisis tend to be relatively open to change. The more narcissistic the patient, however, the more the openness approaches breakdown. Narcissistic defenses are brittle and inflexible and need to be reinforced in order to meet a crisis—it may then be possible for the self to feel protected enough to face facts.

Mr. H was least defended about his work life. He was able to express a range of feelings about the partner who had once been a close friend, and had now betrayed him. But he began to lose objectivity when talking about betrayal, and was more extreme when considering his wife.

Pt: (Furiously.) I have been screwed by my best and closest! These are people I put my trust in.

Th: You've been betrayed by people who should have supported you. [Mirroring to moderate.]

Pt: I've been stabbed in the back!

Th: People who you depended on attacked you, so you protect yourself by going on the attack yourself. [Mirroring interpretation of defensive, externalizing rage.]

Pt: (Mollified.) You said it.

My hope was to acknowledge Mr. H's rage to the point where the actions he must take would not be impetuous and self-destructive. With so much at stake, and the patient so incendiary, it was necessary to "frame" interventions consistently from the patient's point of view:

Pt: That sonofabitch partner of mine thinks he's going to get away with stealing my business. I'll kill him.

Th: I know how serious this betrayal is. But don't you think he'll be expecting just this—for you to be so hurt and angry you'll strike back without concern for yourself?

Pt: Meaning?

Th: Meaning maybe he's counting on your acting before you think.

Pt: Meaning?

Th   Meaning he's counting on your idealism getting in the way of your reason so you'll make a mistake and he'll take advantage of you.

Pt: You're right. I should get off my white horse and think.

At this stage, I simply empathized with his complaints about his children, as I did with his fears of dying. These issues did not take critical priority in the here and now.

3.2.1.5. Short-term treatment

As I continued to mirror Mr. H's grandiosity, he included me in his halo of idealization, and I was able to intensify the interpretive side of my interventions. If I went too far and he attacked, I then emphasized the mirroring of his narcissistic vulnerability. This mended the narcissistic rift, and restored our imagined oneness.

Pt: I'm going to counter-sue this so-called wife until she appreciates what she had with me.

Th: I know she's hurt you, but are you really defending yourself by turning this into World War III?

Pt: What are you saying? I count on you for understanding, and you tell me I'm Saddam Hussein!

Th: So now you feel attacked by me, too.

Pt: What do you mean "feel"—you attacked me!

Th: I hurt you with my lack of understanding. [Mirroring.]

Pt: (mollified.) Damn right.

Th: It pains you when someone you want to value lets you down. You fight back to maintain your rights. [Return to mirroring interpretation.]

Pt: I'll do it for sure.

Th: Maybe it's important to remember sometimes that that reaction plays into the other person's hands.

Pt: I have to remember . . . slow down and remember. I know you're thinking about what's good for me.

The divorce hearing began, and Mr. H found himself constantly humiliated. He responded with anger in court and in his sessions.

Pt: Her and that shyster! They're taking me for a fortune, plus my house.

Th: This is a painful situation. What does your attorney say?

Pt: The son of a bitch tells me I'm lucky she doesn't get a piece of the business.

Th: Husbands can have a rough time in divorce court. Maybe you should play it cool before her demands escalate.

Pt: I know you want the best for me, but are you saying I should give in to this bitch?

Th: You're right. I hope this can work out for you as well as it can. I know it hurts you, but do you think it's in your best interest to challenge the proceedings? Your wife might end up with even more.

Pt: But I hate it! I'll hate myself if I don't fight.

Th: Look—you've already put up a good fight. You want to change the courts, but even your attorney tells you you've reached the limit. You can't keep your money, but you can keep your pride. You can show her she can't get to you.

Pt: That's a lot to ask. Off I go with my tail between my legs.

Th: No. You stand your ground with dignity, whatever insults they hand you. You show your kids that at least one parent has dignity.

Pt: Thank God the kids are on their own.

Th: And they'll appreciate it if their father has the courage not to drag this out, despite the pain.

Pt: It really hurts. I don't know. I don't hear a word from the kids, but maybe this will bring them around.

The divorce proceedings ended as soon as such matters can, primarily because Mr. H decided to hold his temper and keep his dignity. However, he was humiliated by having to move into his own apartment, and worried by the instability of his business. He rapidly transposed his anger from his wife to his partner.

He threatened to take the latter to court, although he himself could ill afford it, and the partner was offering to make a reasonable arrangement. Beneath the anger, Mr

H was suffering from loneliness. It became clear that he needed to set up a fight, not only to ease his humiliation at the divorce, but also to ward off a sense of abandonment. Eventually he extended the projection of his anger into transference acting out when I slipped and tried to reason with him instead of using mirroring interpretation.

Th: Wouldn't it be easier just to stop fighting and accept his offer?

Pt: Are you kidding? I put all my life into this, and I'm going to let this little jerk, this shit take it all away from me? I thought you were on my side.

Th: [Resuming mirroring] I let you down—You don't feel I'm supporting you when you're in a spot.

Pt: Supporting me? God damn it. You and your two-bit degree. What do you know? You're not going through it.

Th: [Persisting] I left you alone when you expected me to be there.

Pt: [Calming down somewhat]. So up yours, doc, with all due respect.

Increasingly mollified by mirroring and mirroring interpretations of his narcissistic vulnerability, the patient settled into a more thoughtful mode.

Pt: At least if my business was going well, I could have some consolation.

Th: It's really tough to tend to the business when you have to deal with your partner, too.

Pt: I feel so lousy—he's betrayed me, and now he wants to settle. I want to see his hide on the wall of my apartment. That's what I'll settle for.

Th: That's a lot of grief for you—to have only the business for your morale, and your partner is ruining it. No wonder you have to stay angry to keep your courage up.

Pt: [Weary and coming around at last] To tell you the truth, the guy can go to hell, but I don't have what it takes to send him there. [Letting go the projection]

Th: Look: you've been fighting hard to defend yourself on all sides, but even the best fighter is going to get disgusted. Nobody else is going to give you a break. You're stuck with your own pain, and all you can do is take it out on yourself.

Pt: I'm coming to a decision. It makes me sick just to hear this guy's voice. I'll compromise for the sake of peace with the bastard.

Th: A tough decision.

Pt: [Very serious] To tell you the truth, sitting in my apartment staring at the T. V. and trying to figure out where I'm going is not for me. But even making a decision feels lousy. Work stinks. My kids don't call. I don't sleep much; I keep thinking about all this crap that has come down—Over and over—and then it's morning.

Th: Tell me some more about that.

Pt: All this—it takes me back, you know—life never was so great.

Th: [Unexpectedly choking up, and realizing it is projective identification] You know, I think there's a lot of sadness here. Do you think you're being tough and covering over your feelings more than you have to?

Pt: [Close to tears] I haven't felt this crummy since I was a kid. Just a snotty little kid alone in my room. Doc, I don't want to go back to that place again.

Mr. H left in a dejected state of mind, and next session reported that he wanted to "get out of this; I think we should call it quits." I replied: "The feelings coming up here are difficult for you. Because the feelings are coming up in the session, you figure you can make them go away by stopping the therapy." [Countering his acting out] He answered: "O.K., O.K. But I don't like where this is going. I'm trusting you to make this come out right." [Re-establishment of idealization]

With the completion of the divorce and settling of matters with his former partner, Mr. H grew increasingly depressed. He still searched for a place to project his anger, and so to ward off the depression. Consequently, he focused on the relationships with his grown children.

Pt: There's no empathy, doc. They're all staying away. All I get is the credit card bills from the little one.

Th: This is hard for you.

Pt: How could they forget everything they got from me—advice, money—they always had the best.

Th: They stay so far away from you, you reassure yourself by recalling all you gave them.

Pt: Someone should remember. Any advice, doc?

Th: It's hard to believe you've run out of ideas.

Pt: Well, I thought about calling—reaching out, you know. But those kids, I spoiled them. How do they know how to give?

Th: You're so disappointed, you shield yourself from possible increased disappointment by assuming their reaction. [Addressing devaluing defense]

Pt: Maybe I should put in a call to my son. He sometimes listens to me.

Mr. H reached out to his children, and was gratified to find them responsive. They had been cautiously waiting for him to make the first move.

Mr. H was not gratified, however, by the increase in his depression after his temporary elation. His anger again turned to me—a risky happening with the narcissist who requires harmony with the idealized therapist. But uncomfortable as this was for both of us, it seemed to show that our relationship was becoming more realistic: transference acting out might be shifting toward a real relationship where transference was not so much the entire interaction as a distortion in it.

Pt: What is this? The more I follow your advice, they worse I feel! I think you better go back to shrink school.

Th: You've got a point. The more progress you make, the more the feelings come out. You've become strong enough to handle what was too painful before.

Pt: Yeah. It's "too painful," and now I'm going to "protect myself" by getting out of here before it gets worse. [Sarcastic demonstration that he is integrating mirroring interpretation]

Th: So I use jargon. Could you ever run your real estate business without talking the talk? The main thing is, since you've been here, you've gone through one crisis after another, and you still have your business and your kids and your pride. You're managing.

Pt: Big gold star! And I sit in this hole of an apartment with my blank walls and my nightmares. My recreation is thinking up ways to kill you slowly.

Th: This is hard work. You've met your practical problems, and now this thing with feelings comes up. Easier to blame me than say this is what you didn't want to experience. [Taking a chance with patient's increased strength to try a mild confrontation]

Pt: You're what I don't want to experience. Like all the others, you have my money, and I have my grief.

Th: It's easier to experience me than experience that grief.

Once again, I felt an unexpected wave of sorrow flood me, and realized I was identifying with his projected sadness. I tried to remain still and neutral, but my nose started to run. As I sniffed and reached in my pocket for a tissue, I said:

"It's really tough when you work so hard and it comes up crap anyway."

My patient put his head in his hands and was silent for many seconds.

Then he said: "It's too much like her. You make me think of my mother. You tell me to spit it out, and then you rub it all over my face."

I waited.

"My mom. She told me all her troubles, but she couldn't listen to mine. 'Tell me one of your jokes,' she'd say. That's how I got to be the God damn life of the party."

We sat together in silence gain.

"Doc, there's things I never talked about to anyone. I don't want to here, either. What's the point?"

"Maybe this will be the toughest decision you make here."

"I don't know. I have to think this one out, maybe next time."

But he did not return to the subject for the next two sessions. Here and now sessions took center stage, and I did not press him. Narcissists tend to be under the pressure of an unacknowledged obligation, and encouragement, however well meant, is perceived as an excess obligation. Mr. H had been in therapy for two and a half years, and was shifting from acting out his issues defensively to examining them realistically despite transference distortion. This transference distortion had led him to trace anger at me to anger at his mother, and now he hesitated on the brink of needed but unwelcome insight.

He said: "After all these years, I have nothing to say to her, so why should I have anything to say to you?"

"Just tell me what you choose to."

He shifted uncomfortably, then looked me in the eye.

"My dad was pretty mean, you know. I didn't tell you, but he slapped me and my brother around some. He slapped my mom around, too. My brother ran and hid, but I always took it, and I stood between him and my mom, too, till he knocked me down.

"When he. slammed out of the house, my mom would put her arms around me. She said: 'Harry, you're my guardian angel.' Then she'd kiss me."

He looked down. "This is the part I don't talk about. She'd kiss me on the mouth and take me to her bed. She used to snuggle me, and we'd stay there a long time.

A silence passed.

"It felt good, but it felt all mixed up."

A quick gesture of dismissal.

"What's the point of this? Let the dead rest."

3.2.1.6. Long-term Therapy

Mr. H had reached an important juncture in his treatment. He had achieved some observing distance with his defenses, and was less inclined to impulsively act out. He had dealt with his critical presenting problems, and had begun to look within himself. And he had established a rapport with me primarily as a real person, rather than an idealized protector or adversary.

For the next several weeks he talked about his childhood—especially about his father's abusive sternness and his devotion to his mother. He also grew increasingly depressed, and dropped the joking facade that had marked the first years of treatment.

Pt: I feel lousy.

Th: Allowing for the unhappiness you feel, it's almost like meeting you for the first time. You know how you said you had to be "the life of the party" to please your mother? Well, it's like I've had to be your straight man to keep things going. We've had to keep the one liners going, you know?

Pt: Yeah. Keep the sunny side up. Never cry in front of mom—she's been through enough.

During his first two years of therapy, Mr. H passed his 61st birthday, the age at which his father had died. The safe navigation of that year, plus the completion of his divorce and settlement with his partner, gave him a sense of relief, but left him with fewer hiding places for his anxiety and depression. He refused medication, although he reported insomnia, angry outbursts, and persistent recollections of his mother's death.

Pt: I keep thinking how she was at the end. She was so
      pale. Her nose and chin were so sharp and she didn't
      recognize me. I can't get rid of this picture. I see myself
      kissing her goodbye and I feel sick. I get this ringing in
      my head. I feel like I'm a little lost kid.

I said very little, not wishing to interrupt the deepening
and flow of his feelings. I also had an uneasy sense that
something was surfacing that had been held down as his
feelings had been held down. One session he took and deep
breath and looked at me earnestly.

He said: "There's more I haven't talked about, doc.
Maybe now is the time to tell someone and get it said." He
hesitated, then continued, "When I was a little kid—when
my dad hit her—she did more than take me to bed. She
used to stroke me, if you get what I'm saying, and she took
it pretty far."

He shook his head slowly: "It was too much like she
needed me even if it wasn't good for me. I think that's why
I always feel like a phony—this important phony who's
someone's favorite toy."

He was silent for a long time, staring ahead of him.

"This is too much, doc, I'm leaving early today."

I did not attempt to confront the pain that seemed
appropriate, and not a characterological bluff.

I said: "Are you sure you want to call it quits for today?
You're talking about some important stuff."

"I really want out. I'll pick it up next time."

I believed he was calling for a necessary pacing, and we
ended the session.

The next several sessions were marked by long silences
interspersed with painful memories that became more
graphic as they came into focus through dreams and verbal

descriptions. He said: "I dreamed I was lying next to mom. It felt like the most wonderful thing in the world. Then this is really tough to say—I came in my sleep. I woke up and hated myself, but you know, even more I hated that I couldn't go back into that dream. Why did she do this to me?"

"I can't tell you that. But don't you think this is a reason you often feel so betrayed by life?"

"Yeah, I do. I feel bad and keep on putting on a show to get the magic back. I'm a phony. It's all false."

Mr. H had always been partly aware of his mother's sexual abuse of him. With his increasing ability to face his feelings, he was also able to face his traumatic memories more clearly. He saw how the sense of sexual longing, being used, and needing to please intertwined traumatically and characterologically. He began to understand why he expected to be the center of attention, yet felt undervalued at the same time.

3.2.1.7. Termination

Mr. H had been in therapy over three years. The sessions slowly became reports of daily events, anecdotes and jokes. I questioned him about this.

Th: Your sessions have changed. It has been painful for you to talk about your past and your mother, but it has helped you to know yourself better.

Pt: It's true. But it's too much. The dreams keep coming, and the sexual feelings, and the nausea. I want to remember my mom differently. I want this to stop.

Th: If you let yourself fully acknowledge the past, it will stop. And you'll be in a better place than before. The bad feelings that have blocked some of the good feelings about your mother will be gone. You'll remember her realistically, but mixed with the love you always had.

Pt: And honestly, how long is this supposed to take?

Th: I can't say. And honestly, it may get worse before it gets better, although it will be better in the end.

Pt: I don't know. I'm not sure I'm looking for this better reality.

Mr. H did not pursue his early trauma. I made certain his choice was a deliberate, conscious one, but he was aware of the path he was taking.

Then one day he came in with his spirits raised.

Pt: Doc, you know I've signed up with this dating service. Would you believe I've struck it rich?

Th: You found someone you like?

Pt: For real! You know how you always said "real" is best? She's no pin-up, but nice. She cooks, she likes the same movies, she helps me talk to my kids!

Th: Sounds like this may be something solid.

Pt: Believe it! And no more bad dreams.

Th: You're truly affectionate?

Pt: Oh, yes. This is love-making. Makes me happy to wake up in the morning, you know?

The weeks passed, and Mr. H began to talk about the possibility of marriage. He was aware that he had made his choice in part to close over the early trauma.

He said: "That was a bad trip. I needed to get it off my chest. But there's no point going back there any more. What's done is done, and it's time to move on.

"Look—my business is O.K., my kids even visit me, and I'm marrying a good woman. I know I used to rub people the wrong way, but I'm more mellow now. And I got good people to set me straight when I stray.

"You got to know I was never made to go it alone. Now I'm complete. Why should I go back there somewhere in a bad past when it's O.K. in the present?"

He stayed a few more sessions but, as he had pointed out, he had resolved his presenting problems, modified his character issues, and found a satisfactory life for himself. The early traumatic issue that had emerged as a result of the strengthening of his personality had been partially dealt with; but it was no longer a secret and was woven into the conscious narrative of his life. His new relationship had offered him a short-cut to resolution, but seemed substantial. Fundamentally, patients know their own limits and tolerances—it is the therapist's job to bring this knowledge as much into awareness as possible. The patient then makes his own choices.

3.3. A Patient with "Closet" Narcissistic Personality Disorder, Recent PTSD, and Developmental Trauma

The basic narcissistic personality disorder was described in the last chapter. Although the "closet" narcissist (as defined by Masterson, 1981, pp. 7-8) seems very different from the manifest or overt narcissist, the underlying dynamic is the same, and should be understood if effective treatment is to take place.

The two conditions seem so different at first, because the overt narcissist defensively devalues the other, while the closet narcissist devalues the self. The goal in either case is to create a sense of idealized merger—either by bringing the self into conformity with the other (closet narcissists are often co-dependents), or by bringing the other into conformity with the self (overt narcissists often make forceful leaders, although they may not be well liked).

As Masterson notes, the closet narcissist presents as inhibited and even ineffective, only to reveal grandiose dynamics in the course of the treatment. These dynamics are foreshadowed by a perfectionism and stubbornness that seem impervious to intervention, and frustrate the therapist. The patient may ask for advice and appear dependent on the therapist's "wisdom," but basically takes a self-determined tack and will not budge from it. So the closet narcissist initially seems to be a compliant, "easy" patient, who later turns out to be fixed in self-focused ways that may be maladaptive, but are well-armored against change.

Like manifest narcissism, closet narcissism probably has its origins in mother-child interpersonal dysfunction in the practicing sub-phase of separation-individuation. During the sub-phase, there is a mutual mirroring and sense of oneness that supports the child's pleasure in exploration of the surrounding world. The outgoing child for awhile experiences the mother as an internal part of the self, and "borrows" her imagined omnipotence. When the illusion wears thin, the child returns to the mother to renew the sense of oneness and invulnerability.

Too much distance, over-possessiveness, or inconsistency in the mother-child interaction can lead to insecurity or over-reliance in the practicing child.

Like the manifest narcissist, the closet narcissist lives in an inner world of sharply divided "good" and "bad" (part) objects. The closet narcissist is as dedicated to maintaining an idealized relationship, but keeps it going by compliance and even self-sacrifice. When these maneuvers do not gain the required approval, the closet narcissist often reacts with righteous indignation. This anger can be unrelenting unless the hurt that underlies is acknowledged, and the rift in the sense of idealized oneness is repaired.

Manifest and closet narcissism both rely on *idealization* as a major defense. The difference is that the manifest narcissist demands idealization from others, while the closet narcissist will *devalue the self* and rationalize the shortcomings of the other in order to keep the other on a pedestal. If the indignation of the closet narcissist is not met with mirroring of the pain, the closet narcissist will *detach* from the other rather than tolerate the introduction of ambivalent or negative feelings into the relationship.

Both types of narcissistic personality disorder share the following defenses with the borderline: *acting out, splitting, projective identification, projection, denial,* and *avoidance.*

Mirroring Interpretation of Narcissistic Vulnerability: This intervention was described in the previous chapter. Briefly, Masterson describes this as a means of therapeutic communication that by-passes the narcissist's antipathy to interpretation; the narcissist's sense of vulnerability is mirrored, and defenses are acknowledged for their capacity for self-protection. The intervention at first shows understanding for feelings of pain; and then the need of the self for protection against the pain; and finally, non-critical identification of the defense mechanism the self uses to ward off or mask the pain.

This formula of "pain . . . self . . . defense" is applied to maladaptive defenses in the following examples of intervention:

Idealization (of the other): "You find it so painful to accept your husband's failure to work, that you protect yourself by saying the available jobs are beneath him."

Devaluation (of the self): "You are so distressed by your husband's rudeness, you protect yourself by holding yourself responsible."

Detachment: "You have been deeply hurt, and you are trying to soothe yourself by withdrawing from the situation."

Acting out: "I think this session is causing you distress, and you hope to dilute the situation by cancelling next week."

Projective Identification: I sense a tension in the atmosphere—could it be that you are not fully aware of your stress because it would be uncomfortable for you?"

Projection: "I wonder if it hurts so much to see your responsibility it this matter, that you protect yourself by seeing your boss as wholly at fault. "

Denial:	"It's so unpleasant to think your boss might disagree with you, that you try to keep things smooth by pretending there isn't a problem."
Avoidance:	"The topic we were just discussing is a painful one for you, so you protect yourself by changing the subject."

(Mirroring alone, without interpretation, may be necessary at times when the patient feels especially vulnerable. *Eg:* "You are very hurt. You sound angry, but I believe you are really feeling misunderstood." Eventually, the mirroring acts as a transition to mirroring interpretation. It must be kept in mind that the narcissist will only make initial progress when feeling understood.)

3.3.1. Case Illustration

Mrs. Clara M composed herself neatly in the chair across from me. She was petite, with a plain, polished appearance that diminished the prettiness of her small features and trim body. Her light brown hair was shaped into a shiny helmet. She wore freshly-pressed jeans and white shirtwaist, with old but freshly-whitened sneakers, She wore a touch of lipstick, and no jewelry other than a wrist-watch and a wedding band. Her manner was politely-spoken, and attentive to the point of deference.

She was in her early forties, with a husband in the construction business, and four children—two in their early twenties and independent, and two teen-agers. She maintained a freelance day-care service, and, until recently, had been leading an active, demanding life in her community. She had had no previous experience with therapy, and was very much a believer that problems could be resolved by constructive actions.

3.3.1.1. Presenting problem

Nearly a year ago, Mrs. M had experienced a traumatic accident. A child had suddenly run in front of the car she was driving and, to avoid hitting the child, Mrs. M swerved into an oncoming car. No one was seriously injured, although there was damage to both vehicles, and Mrs. M suffered from whiplash. The pain in Mrs. M's neck and back persisted, even after there were no medical findings, and healing was assumed to have taken place. Her sleep was disturbed, as well, and she hesitated to drive—she would avoid the necessity or accept it with anxiety and a tendency to overreact to routine actions of pedestrians or other drivers. Her physician had referred her for psychotherapy, and Mrs. M had complied, but took offense: "He's saying my back is in my head," she told me resentfully.

3.3.1.2. History

Mrs. M's family history, like herself, was presented as orderly and uneventful. Her mother was still living: a church-going widow devoted to good works. However, her parents had divorced when the patient was four years old, although the patient had never been clear about the reason.

The mother had remarried to a reclusive man who related marginally to the patient and to the sister who came from this second marriage. The step-father died of a heart attack when the patient was married and pregnant with her fourth child.

Mrs. M's own marriage went smoothly. She was attentive to her husband, who was a good provider.

Her boys, 23 and 16 years old, did well, relating warmly to their extraverted father. The girls were slightly more problematic. Mrs. M tended to be overprotective of them, so that the 19-year-old had moved out somewhat prematurely, and the 13-year-old tended to cling to her mother.

Aside from the experience of her step-father's death, Mrs. M's life had been marked by a former, possibly traumatic event. In her early 'teens, she had seen her best friend struck by a car. Fortunately, the damage had been limited to a broken arm, but Mrs. M had been horrified, and blamed herself for calling her friend's name and distracting her. Mrs. M was aware of the probability of some subjective connection between this early happening and her recent accident, but never took this from the intellectual to the emotional realm. "Bad things happen," she said, "and so do bad coincidences." She seemed to tuck the matter away, but I noticed she kept turning the ring on her finger, and that her hands were shaking.

3.3.1.3. Introductory phase

Although she continued to tend to her responsibilities, Mrs. M did so with effort, a sense of stress, and physical pain. Her back was worse whenever she tended the children in her care (Lively three to five year olds), and she had to invent games and activities that minimized picking the children up or running after them. She admitted this was a lost cause, and refused to take pain-killers for fear of becoming inattentive.

She did show initiative by getting her husband to agree to complete the fencing-in of the property.

Pt: But he's so busy, he just doesn't get to it.

Th: I think it pains you to ask for extra help, so you protect yourself by being extra patient.

Pt: It's so. My husband is such a busy man. I hate to nag him.

Th: Is it nagging to give him an opportunity to give you a hand?

Pt: Well, I just don't like to make demands for myself.

Th: Isn't your husband concerned with your well being?

Pt: Of course he is! That helps me keep my troubles to myself.

Th: Seems to me you're between a rock and a hard place: it pains you to ask for help, but even you may be overwhelmed by this extra stress, and end up worrying him.

Pt: Well, perhaps I might remind him after supper.

Th: Why not? As you say, he's busy and just needs a reminder.

Pt: Come to think of it, he did ask me to keep reminding him.

Th: Of course. And think how much better you'll both feel knowing it's impossible for any child to run into the street.

Pt: It would be a weight off my mind.

She followed through, and her husband responded with admirable speed. Were there any other issues of daily functioning that could be resolved? She was afraid to back the car out of the garage, to the point that her husband had to do it before going to work. She was afraid some neighbor's child might be out of sight behind her vehicle. Again, the husband's skills were called upon.

Th: Could he install a back-up signal like the ones they have on trucks?

Pt: I hate to trouble him when he's so busy. And he just did me a favor with the fence.

Th: I think your husband likes to please you and show his competence. But it discomforts you so much to ask for help that you try to comfort yourself by being stoical.

Pt: Well, it does inconvenience him to back my car out every morning. Perhaps if he just took the one time to install something, it would be easier for him overall.

It was becoming clear to me that Mrs. M had a diagnosis of probable PTSD and closet narcissistic personality disorder. The PTSD was evidenced in her mixed avoidance and persistent anxiety about driving; her hypervigilance about pedestrians (when she was driving), or of children running into the road (during her day-care sessions); her persistent recollections of the accident that kept her awake at night; her selective back pain; and the fact that she was still troubled by these symptoms nearly a year after the accident.

The closet narcissism was suggested by her protective idealization of her husband, whom she considered too important to be bothered by her reasonable requests; her consistent placing of the needs of others before her own; her approval-seeking perfectionism to the point of self-devaluation; and her responsiveness to mirroring interpretations of her narcissistic vulnerability. Like many closet narcissists, she placed doing and protecting before her own feelings (especially about herself).

In turn, I became aware of typical countertransference reactions she induced in me, such as an impatient wish to get things done (probably a reflection of her expectation that I would, like her mother, take a no-nonsense approach to doing the "right thing"). When I wasn't inclined to push her, I found myself engulfed by a sense of helplessness, which I believe was her projective identification of her own unacceptable feeling.

With her husband's help, Mrs. M had eased some of her practical problems. She was somewhat less frozen in the fear of letting another get hurt, saw me as a sensible ally, and began to speak more freely.

3.3.1.4. Initial Psychotherapy

With starts and stops, Mrs. M was encouraged to tell me in detail about the accident. Sometimes she seemed relieved to tell another person. Sometimes she was inclined to avoid it: a mixture of her PTSD and her belief that she was complaining too much.

Pt: Should I be indulging myself like this?

Th: It's an important part of your therapy to put into words—as much as you can—what happened.

Pt: But I already told you what happened. So did Dr. Q [the referring doctor] in his letter.

Th: It's difficult for you to dwell on a subject that touches your feelings—I think you try to save yourself discomfort by dismissing the matter.

Pt: Well, if you think it'll help, I'll go over it again. [Defending by idealizing me/devaluing her]

Th: Is it hard for you to see the advantage to yourself? [Pushing on the defense too much]

Pt: I'm willing to do this if you think it will help you to find the answers to my problems. [Remains defended despite agreement to continue]

She described what had happened. She had backed her car out of the garage and turned it into the street. Suddenly, a ball came rolling from between parked cars. Sure enough, a little girl, about seven, dashed after the ball. Mrs. M knew she couldn't stop in time, and swerved into the oncoming lane. As bad luck would have it, another car was approaching and they collided—more luckily, at low speeds. Mrs. M was stunned, then horrified, when she could no longer see the child. She and the other driver, a man, shakily got out of their vehicles and together hurried toward the sound of a child crying in terror. They found the little girl where she had lost her balance and fallen next to the passenger side of Mrs. M's car. Mrs. M felt close to fainting—sounds were distant and tinny—but the man took her arm reassuringly. "Thank God no one was hurt." Then he took out a cell phone and began to call 911 to bring the police. Thank God," he repeated, "we won't need any paramedics."

At this point, a woman, undoubtedly the child's mother, ran from a nearby house. She saw her child sitting on the ground and dashed to her. Then she started screaming at Mrs. M, accusing her of nearly killing her little girl. Mrs. M continued to feel distant and increasingly detached; she stared at the woman.

The man came to her defense, pointed to the ball, asked the mother where was *she,* anyway? Soon the police arrived and methodically took control of the situation.

"I couldn't sleep for a week. I kept seeing the little girl running toward the car. Over and over. I couldn't stop the picture from playing over and over in my head. And the terror in the child's voice! And the mother screaming accusations! And I kept thinking I could have killed that little girl, or how I could have hurt that man. I couldn't drive for weeks, and I couldn't take the car out of the driveway at all. And then my back! I couldn't lie back or sit myself up for a week, and after that, it acted up every time I tried to sit in the car seat. I've had x-rays, and scans, and the doctor says I should be all right, but I can't drive without pain. And I can't drive without the fear it'll happen all over again."

Mrs. M was convinced her problem could be "fixed" through her own will power, medication, or possibly hypnosis (she was skeptical, but Dr. Q had suggested it). She had gone as far as will power would take her; an antidepressant and a minor tranquilizer (which was also a muscle relaxer) eased her somewhat and facilitated her sleeping. She agreed to give hypnosis a try, and I helped her to juxtapose images of calm with the traumatic scenes to a slight benefit. I also helped her to transfer some of the back pain to her left foot (once I was clear physical sources of the pain had been ruled out). But all these interventions only served to modify the problem. I was increasingly convinced Mrs. M's traumatic reaction might have past antecedents that should be explored.

Th: I know that what happened was very frightening to you. I also know you have conscientiously done everything you could think of to remedy the situation. One thing we really haven't explored is how what happened might have stirred up something in your past.

Pt: Now you're saying, like Dr. Q, it's all in my mind.

Th: I'm saying that what effects us emotionally effects the entire self: think of how people get colds when they're stressed out. Think of how people suffer headaches from tension. [Taking a cognitive approach to meet a defense that appears to arise from trauma rather than character]

Pt: Now you're saying "I'm making it up." [Continued denial]

Th: No, your pain is real. But I think it causes you more distress to think the pain begins in your feelings, because you believe feelings can be controlled by will, and you can't control them. So you push away the idea that pain can come from feelings. [Speaking to her characterological sense of vulnerability again]

Pt: Of course we control our feelings! What would happen if we didn't?

Th: We control how we *act* on our feelings. Feelings themselves come and go like weather.

[Return to the cognitive—to clarify distortion in reasoning]

Pt: I never thought of it like that. I just feel so helpless to stop my fears. [Some concession in response to alternating interventions]

Mrs. M finally conceded that she had been persistently troubled by memories of her teen-age friend being struck by a car. But she had decided it was an indulgence to be bothered this way by something that had already happened. Comments to the effect that seemingly finished business should not be disturbing her, did not touch her no-nonsense characterological stance.

Pt: What's done is done. I've no business wallowing in the past.

Th: It's painful looking back at things you can't change. You feel more at case setting them aside.

Pt: It is painful and I just can't see the point in it.

Th: It's possible you could surprise yourself and find it helpful, but the discomfort of reviewing the past is something you can guarantee. So you avoid it to stay on the safe side.

Pt: Well, if you really think so . . . I'll try. I'll rely on your knowledge.

Th: [Feeling a strong countertransference urge to shake the patient] Does it feel so unprotected to explore for yourself?

Pt: (Sighing and smiling slightly) I suppose if I'm here to try everything, I should have the courage to do it.

Mrs. M lowered her defenses and talked of the past. She had just turned thirteen when she saw her best friend struck by a car. He friend was crossing the street when Clara waved and called to her from the far sidewalk. A car making a sudden right turn on the red light failed to brake in time, and the friend did not see the car until it knocked her down, breaking her arm in the fall Clara rushed to her friend, but was soon pushed aside by adults who came to help.

Afterward, no one—including the friend—blamed her in any way, but no one talked to her about her unhappiness, either. She lost sleep and lost weight. Her mother took her for B12 shots, and Clara kept her shame to herself.

Pt: I could have killed her.

Th: What a difficult situation for a thirteen-year old! You were excited to see your friend, who was crossing the street with the light. How could you have acted more naturally? [Cognitive]

Pt: I don't know why she wasn't angry with me.

Th: Exchange places. Supposing she had called out to you while you were crossing with the light and didn't see the car coming around the corner? Would you have blamed *her*? [Cognitive]

Pt: [Remaining in defense] I probably would have blamed myself.

Th: Why? You had the right of way, didn't you? What did the police say? [Still cognitive]

Pt: I found out later they gave the driver a summons.

Th: So the police held the driver responsible—not either of you.

Pt: I feel a little better. Maybe I've been too hard on myself.

Th: Sometimes it's easier to see an emotional situation when you look from other people's point of view.

Pt: Yes. I see a scared teen-ager with no adult to reassure her.

She conceded, after this cognitive exchange, that being able to recount this event, even years later, was a relief. And she felt there was a correspondence between this and the recent happening. Both times, she had felt the horror and helplessness of facing the impending accident, and the wrenching sense of guilt afterwards.

Surprisingly, she followed this achievement with the announcement that she thought it was time to leave therapy. The personality disorder triad apparently had been touched off, and I tried to explain this to her.

"Sometimes. when things get clearer to a patient, they feel they are somehow stepping into forbidden territory, and try to withdraw. Follow the sense of relief you had at first, and see if you might want to stay with it awhile longer."

She agreed to stay, but, for the first time, faced me directly with her frustration at trying to drive, and her continued back pain. What was the point in it all, if these symptoms could not be relieved. No doubt this was not my fault, but what was the point?

I felt diminished, and told myself the feeling was induced as a by-product of her own helplessness.

Then I persisted, looking for a way to connect constructively with her pain.

Her concern for her thirteen-year-old daughter began to take center stage. The patient could not let her daughter enter a car—including the family car—without extreme anxiety. She became angry when I saw through this as a projection of her own unresolved concerns.

Pt: Why are you making me feel like some neurotic? A daughter's health is a mother's concern.

Of course you have a right to be concerned. [Mirroring] But isn't it possible that keeping your daughter home shelters you from the pain of recalling your own experience? [Mirroring interpretation]

Th: Of course you have a right to be concerned. [Mirroring] But isn't it possible that keeping your daughter home shelters you from the pain of recalling your own experience? [Mirroring interpretation]

Pt: My daughter is too happy-go-lucky. She doesn't know what's out there. And you don't know a mother's feelings.

I thought my interventions were going nowhere, until I found that Mrs. M had sat down with her daughter and husband, discussed the situation, and learned that they thought she was being overprotective.

She flipped back her bangs with her hand, set her jaw, and said:

"I've overdone it. I have to continue here so I won't take out my anxieties on my family."

She paused, then looked at me earnestly:

"Are you still there for me? I wasn't kind to you."

I assured her that I thought she had acted well, and that I expected her to voice all her feelings in therapy. To cover all the bases, I added the mirroring interpretation that sometimes, when she saw her worries reflected in the actions of another, she tried to calm herself by modifying her worries by proxy.

3.3.1.5. Long-term treatment

A new, long-term phase of therapy opened after the first two years of treatment. Mrs. M was functioning well, had loosened her anxious grip on her daughter, and was more direct with her husband.

She showed a fuller sense of separateness, allowing herself to have differences with others, including myself.

Her ability to express and resolve anger at me showed the beginning of a therapeutic alliance.

But the presenting issues persisted. She was still fearful of driving, even though she did so regularly, and her back hurt her whenever she took the driver's seat. Although she continued to do useful character work, improving her relationships within the family, she became increasingly frustrated, even irritable about her persisting anxiety and backaches when driving.

I approached her tentatively—first trying to resolve characterological resistances, acknowledging she must be disappointed at the lack of progress around the presenting issues.

Pt: Yes. I'm frustrated. I feel something else is there.

I found myself in a more direct mode, trying to search out traumatic issues that might have been missed.

Pt: I often wonder if there's something there. I keep dreaming over and over of a little girl being killed. When I wake up, I'm haunted by it.

I asked her if there were family members who could fill in more of her history. At first she demurred, then changed her mind as her dreams became more vivid.

Pt: I dreamed I looked at the child who had been killed. She had my face! I woke my husband up when I screamed.

With encouragement from her husband, she decided to approach her step-sister (child of her mother's second

115

husband). They were not close, but there had always seemed to be a bond of unspoken understanding between them.

The response was evocative. The half-sister told her she should ask her mother, and to return to her if she found no answer. Mrs. M quickly visited her mother, who became nervous when questioned, and denied any secret knowledge. Further provoked by her mother's defensiveness, Mrs. M returned to the half sister, who silently handed her a photograph of three-to-four-year-old twin sisters sitting in a double stroller. Then the half-sister told her the family secret.

Mrs. M turned frantically to me.

Pt: You never told me the past could hide such things! I feel as if my reality is crumbling. It looks like I had a twin sister and my father ran over her! That's horrible . . . worse to live with than not knowing. Why didn't you prepare me?

I acknowledged her shock and disorientation, but also reflected that the only person who could have prepared her for the loss of a twin sister was her mother. I suggested that her feelings needed to be directed toward her mother, who had withheld her own history from her.

Mrs. M became calmer and determined to confront her mother. She wasted no time (like most closet narcissists, she was a doer), and soon her mother broke down and admitted that, in a tragic accident, her first husband had backed his car over the sister while little Clara had watched (although she had been amnestic for the entire episode). The mother divorced her husband—she could not bear the sight of him—he disappeared from their lives completely, and the mother remarried. Her mother had told her second husband of her reason for divorcing, and had refused to discuss the matter thereafter. Similarly, after telling Mrs. M this much, the mother refused to discuss things further. Mrs. M was furious, and accused her mother of robbing her of her past—even of taking away a part of herself. But the mother turned away, and had nothing more to say.

Mrs. M returned to her half-sister, who further clarified that her father had given her the photo with the instructions she show it to Mrs. M if she should ever ask about her unspoken past. The step-father had never agreed with the mother to keep the past a secret, but honored her wishes to a point.

For a week or two, Mrs. M seemed relieved and satisfied. I thought she had made a critical breakthrough that might, in time, be reflected in the lightening of her symptoms. Instead, she became increasingly disturbed, and again threatened to drop out of therapy.

Pt: My whole life is changed. I hate my mother. Why didn't you advise me to leave it alone? I am so angry that you have burdened me with this impossible past.

Th: [Deciding to go with the patient's vulnerability] Therapy seems to have brought you more problems than you started with. I should have made you more aware of what you could have opened up. How can you find a way to feel less hurt? [Mirroring]

Pt: I'm so upset. My life is crazy. How can you help me change the past? I've always done the right thing, and still bad things happen. They happen whenever I start to feel confident. It just isn't fair.

Th: [Switching somewhat to a cognitive response] Because you are there when something happens, or you get upsetting information when you reach out, doesn't mean you caused any of it. You have an unusual and difficult past, but knowing about it, no matter how painful, helps you put your life in one piece. There are fewer shadows.

Pt: Maybe so. I want to trust what you say. But I feel unprepared for all of this. Therapy makes me sick.

The impasse continued, until I said: "You feel deeply injured because your mother has refused to confide in you, and you cannot feel protected by your mutual understanding. She looked silently at the floor, and had difficulty speaking any further in that session. My mirroring interpretation of her narcissistic vulnerability had touched upon the abandonment depression and relieved it somewhat.

Mrs. M began a concentrated confrontation of her mother. The mother, with equal determination, closed her out. Finally, Mrs. M shouted at her mother that her mother didn't care for herself any more than she cared for her dead sister, and might as well forget her. The mother burst out defensively, saying the subject was too overwhelming, but adding that she still loved her daughter.

Pt: What can I do? My mother can't get beyond her own misery. She has no time for me.

Th: Perhaps this is one more difficult reality you have to face, at least for now. But perhaps if you face it, you can put some things to rest. And perhaps time will bring a change.

Over the weeks, the patient's resentment of her mother abated, giving way to a deep grief that reached beyond the mother to the patient's whole history, especially the loss of a sister. She wept that she had experienced much misfortune, and had suffered helplessly because she didn't know what she was suffering from. Her anger at therapy and me faded, as she took back her defensive projection and began to accept a realistic view of her life.

She cried in sessions; she cried at home. At last, she was crying for herself.

For the next year, Mrs. M journeyed through the deep grief work that lies at the heart of both character and trauma work. Beyond separation anxiety and the fear of remembering, lies the profound sadness that dissolves the frozen core of the self.

It was clear that Mrs. M was finding herself in the maze of her being when she discovered she was driving more spontaneously and with less pain.

"How can it be?" she asked. "The more pain I face, the less pain I feel!" She had both strengthened herself and traveled through traumatic recollections known and "unknown," and had emerged a more complete and assertive person.

Mrs. M was able to accept her mother's distance for what it was, and separate it from her general relationship with her mother. This empathic move kept their relationship intact and showed her advance to real relationship. But the two could never be as close again, and Mrs. M would never trust entirely the things her mother told her.

3.4. A Patient with Schizoid Personality Disorder, recent PTSD, and Developmental Trauma

The Masterson Approach was expanded to include the schizoid personality disorder through the contributions of Ralph Klein, M.D. (1993, 1995). He points out that the *Diagnostic and Statistical Manual* definition of schizoid personality disorder relates to a lower-level state (". . . a pattern of detachment from social relationships and a restricted range of social expression," *DSM IV* p. 629). He holds that the definition of avoidant personality disorder comes closer to describing the higher-level schizoid (". . . a pattern of social inhibition, feelings of inadequacy, and hypersensitivity to negative evaluation, *DSM IV* p. 629). DSM, once again, is descriptively useful, but needs to be anchored in ". . . the nature of the original developmental disturbance, the resultant intrapsychic structure, and the therapeutic manifestation of these features . . ." (Klein, 1993, p. 39).

- *Developmental considerations:* The schizoid personality disorder, according to Klein, was treated not as an individual family member, but as a "dehumanized, depersonified 'function'" of the family. The schizoid speaks of feeling like "an android, a puppet, or a slave" (1993, pp. 40-41).
- *Intrapsychic structure:* The inner world of this patient is divided into two split defensive object relations states, which Klein describes as the "master-slave unit" and the "sadistic-object-self-in-exile unit." The first type of relationship is settled for because it is believed to be "the only condition of relatedness open." The second, which considers others too dangerous to relate to, seeks

safety in "exile," or isolation, at the expense of profound aloneness (pp. 42-43).

- *Defenses:* "Fantasy and self-sufficiency" are "'schizoid compromises'"—efforts to regulate the swings between defensive states and avoid the abandonment depression (pp. 42-43).

- *Therapeutic considerations:* The transference acting out of the schizoid personality disorder follows the intrapsychic structure. The therapist is "placed" in a controlling position, while the patient is resigned to a subordinate state.

Or the therapist is seen as threatening, while the patient retreats to distance and fantasy (pp. 43-44).

> "The key word to describe the nature of the therapeutic alliance here is 'safety,'" and the therapist, carefully maintaining a neutral position, uses *interpretation of the schizoid dilemma* as the primary intervention. As Klein describes it: "The schizoid dilemma is that the patient can be neither too close nor too far in emotional distance from another person without experiencing conflict and anxiety . . . . The therapist's interpretation . . . allows the patient to feel understood and safe" (p. 44).

Klein introduces a second critical intervention—that of the *schizoid compromise.* After the long work of establishing the therapeutic alliance, the patient faces the painful challenge of the abandonment depression. "Here the therapist must look for all signs of defense and resistance and interpret the patient's willingness to 'settle' or 'compromise' on a relatively safe and comfortable distance without working through the abandonment depression" (p. 44).

- *Additional thoughts:* Dr. Klein (1995, pp. 33-43) devotes a chapter to *Developmental Theory,* applying this to the schizoid disorder of the self. Appropriately, Klein argues for not fitting the patient into a developmental "straight jacket;" for not coordinating "dimension[s] of psychopathology . . . with developmental levels" (p. 41).

Without forcing an exact correlation, I believe it is still useful to find parallels between the Mastersonian categories of personality disorder and what might go awry during Mahler's substages of separation/individuation. It must be remembered that people with personality disorders are not small children, but people old enough to use characteristics of past developmental phases as a defensive refuge from psychic pain. Thus, the borderline tolerates both "good" and "bad" feelings, but, like the child of rapprochement, cannot synthesize them.

The narcissist, like the practicing sub-phase child, depends on the maintenance of "good" feelings, and feels annihilated by the presence of "bad." The schizoid, more like the differentiating sub phase child, has little interest in either kind of feeling compared to the emerging realization of the existence of a mother different from the self. Thus, the schizoid personality disorder focuses on degrees of closeness and separation from the other, and has learned to delegate feelings to the realm of fantasy, or such "benign" things as inanimate objects, pets, or ideas. The basic lack of the schizoid is to unite the world of people with the world of feelings. Fantasy in the schizoid (unlike the schizophrenic) does not divide the real from the unreal, but relations with others from expression, even awareness, of directly-related feeling. Probably it is a failure of the mother-child dyad to validate the child's growing sense of a unique, feeling self that sets the stage for schizoid personality disorder later on.

Although all personality disorders have traveled all stages of development (however superficially), only to regress defensively under stress, it is the schizoid who seems most divided by this process. Schizoids may be highly developed in intellectual ability and fund of knowledge, and may even display a quick intuitive grasp of another's character. But there is a fundamental lack of empathy that seems based on a general inhibition of interpersonal feeling—a feeling which is not missing, but is relegated to a very private world hedged about by acute sensitivity to interpersonal hurt. As Klein points out, "safety" is a critical issue for the schizoid. This personality disorder is the most elusive to work with because the sense of basic trust is the most difficult to build with him or her.

Interventions with the schizoid rely on their strong intellectual defenses. In addition to the interpretation of the schizoid dilemma and of the schizoid compromise, I would add that schizoid patients are often receptive to interventions directed to their preoccupation with puzzling things out. A patient of mine who was clever at investing in the stock market, but frightened of buying a new house, reacted positively when I pointed out the similarities in researching both markets.

The impasse was broken when the patient was able to see buying a house as an intellectual exercise rather than an emotion-laden commitment to his family.

In my experience, schizoid patients also respond well to mirroring interpretations—not so much of their sense of vulnerability, but of their sense of danger. The formula for this intervention then becomes: mirror the sense of risk; affirm the need to keep the self safe; then describe objectively the means of defense. ("Going to the party feels risky to you, so you protect yourself by staying home where you feel safe."

Although schizoid patients move slowly (cautiously) in therapy, higher-level patients, because of their strong intellectual defenses, may seem to move more quickly initially. Because of their interest in figuring things out and piecing them together, they may make good progress in defining their maladaptive patterns of behavior and defense. As Klein describes, it is the crossing over to the therapeutic alliance, and the opening up to the abandonment depression that pose the greatest therapeutic challenge.

The ability of the patient to negotiate these transitions marks the difference between short and long-term treatment. The schizoid shares many early defenses with other personality disorders: *acting-out, splitting, projective identification, projection, denial,* and *avoidance.* In addition, the schizoid makes use of *self-sufficiency,* and *fantasy* (Klein, 1993, pp. 43-44).

The following are examples of interventions directed to these defenses as used by the schizoid personality disorder:

Self-sufficiency: "You maintain yourself at a distance from others because it eases the discomfort you have when you move closer."

Fantasy:

"You feel tempted to join in with others, but you feel safer keeping your distance. So you take a half-way position by creating a world of your own where you can set the distances wherever you like."

Acting out:

"You expressed more feeling in this session, so I wonder if you feel at a safer distance by asking to cancel next week."

Splitting:

"Last week you seemed to be talking more freely with me. Today you find it hard to say anything. Do you think you could be shifting to a different mode of relationship because you felt too close?"

Projective Identification:

"It seems to me the mood here has become tense. Do you suppose it might have been because we were talking about feelings, and, in some way, this seems risky to you?"

Projection:

"You tell me that I'm being critical of you, and are drawing away. Could it be that this is how you handle feeling critical of me for asking so many questions?"

Denial:

"It seems to me that you must feel uncomfortable with one foot ready to enter, and the other foot ready to pull back. Perhaps it seems simpler to say there is no problem. "

Avoidance:	"It must seem risky to tell me your thoughts here, so I wonder if you let yourself off the hook by changing the subject."

3.4.1. Case illustration

Charlie Z, 55 and single, worked as a computer technician. He was an only child, whose father had died of a heart attack when the son was fourteen. Mr. Z lived alone, but was attentive to his aging mother, who stayed in an assisted living facility. Of medium build and slender, he presented himself as reserved and almost uniformly grey. Greying at the temples and pale, he wore grey slacks and a white shirt, a grey and brown tweed jacket with leather patches at the elbows, and loafers without tassles. He had a reticent expression, but there was intelligence in his eyes—he was watchful and observant, but sad. He wore no jewelry other than a serviceable watch. He had a careful, serious manner of speaking; when emotional subjects were approached, he dropped into silence, or changed the subject.

3.4.1.2. Presenting problem

Mr. Z had been in his apartment, seated at his computer, when a man with a gun entered the window that opened on the fire-escape. The intruder ordered him into a closet, and pistol-whipped him into unconsciousness. Mr. Z was locked in the closet while his apartment was searched and vandalized. His computer monitor was smashed.

Afterwards, while his bruises were healing, he was emotionally immobilized, and could not return to freelancing for over a month, when necessity forced him into motion. He bought a new computer, and installed a lockable metal grid over the window. He tried to put the memories away from him, but they pressed in over and over. In frequent nightmares, he relived the experience. He played the radio all the time for distraction. He was afraid to leave his apartment, but even more afraid to re-enter it. He kept his reactions to himself, but finally went to his doctor for medication. A minor tranquilizer eased his panic and helped his sleep, while an antidepressant helped his pessimistic state of mind. The doctor also urged him to seek therapy, and at last Mr. Z complied.

3.4.1.3. Short-Term Treatment

Mr. Z approached me diffidently and politely. He took a seat and was silent for awhile. I guessed that his anxiety level was too high to be therapeutic, and offered a business-like structure to the session.

Th: What brings you here, Mr. Z?

Pt: [Uncomfortably] I don't know, really, why I was referred here. What happened is over.

Th: Did the doctor explain why he referred you?

Pt: He said my symptoms could be improved by talking about them.

Th: What are the symptoms?

Pt: I have nightmares; people startle me; I'm uneasy in my apartment; I can't stop thinking about what happened.

Th: Can you tell me what it was that happened?

Pt: Yes.

Th: Please tell me, then, so I can understand the situation more clearly.

Mr. Z gave me a brief, superficial narrative of the event. His voice was matter-of-fact until he came to being locked in the closet—his voice shook then, but he continued. I made a note of his manner, but did not comment.

Th: It sounds as if you have had a very frightening experience.

Pt: [Reluctantly] It was very frightening at the time.

Th: [Experimentally] I wonder if talking about it brings that fear back—perhaps you feel safer letting it alone.

Pt: Frankly, that's what I think. Going through it once was enough. [Silence]

Mr. Z sat stiffly, in a way that made me think his anxiety level had remained high, and he was pulling away. I shifted to more general history-taking.

Mr. Z remained somewhat reluctant, but responded to the telling of his history with less paralyzing anxiety than before. He had been a lonely child. His parents treated him as an adult, and expected him to act like one. He had a hard time relating to other children, and didn't play their games. He explained that, since his parents expected him to know how to act, he hadn't realized that learning was a process. So when he struck out at his first turn at bat, he concluded he was unable to play baseball and gave up. He followed his father around the house, and there he did learn by watching his father's mechanical expertise at carpentry, plumbing, and electrical work. He himself became skilled at figuring how things worked, and at fixing them. Eventually, this led his to his absorption in the technology of computers.

Pt: Computers have their own logic. If you stay with that, they're easy to work with.

Th: You like to puzzle out the nature of a thing?

Pt: Yes.

Th: It could be you would find therapy interesting, then. Therapy is about finding patterns in things, and reasons for things.

Pt: [Hesitantly] I feel the pain.

Th: That's the paradox of psychotherapy. As you figure things out, you have to recreate them, and so, of course, there are feelings that come with that. But you guide yourself with your intellect, which contains and orders those feelings and makes sense of them. But it still comes down to feeling the feelings in order to master them. [Taking a rational and educative approach because the patient's anxiety level has been brought to an exceptional height by his traumatic experience added to an already shy personality]

Pt: [After a silence] I don't know. It still isn't clear to me why I have to feel worse to feel better.

Th: Of course not! You just finished telling me how you were never trained to understand process—you have had to teach yourself [Continued appeal to patient's rational defenses, which seem to help him feel characterologically "safer," combined with cognitive approach, which eases the anxiety connected with PTSD].

Pt: What you say makes me think. But I'm asking a lot of myself. I don't know about this "process." I would like to feel better, but I know—after this discussion today—when I go home, it's going to be harder to get through the front door—things are stirred up.

Th: It sounds as if you're undecided. As if you have one foot half-way in the door, but don't want to give up the reassurance of being still half-way out the door. [Deciding to interpret the schizoid dilemma]

Pt: That's about how it is. These symptoms are in my way, but I don't want to stir up my memories.

Th: So take some time to decide. Suppose you come back for a few sessions—familiarize yourself with the process. Then you'll take it from there.

Pt: I'll think about it and give you a call. Will this time be open if I give you an advance call?

Th: Just call me at least 24 hours in advance. If the time is open, it's yours. Otherwise, we'll reschedule.

Following Klein's guidelines, I gave Mr. Z enough space to feel he was safe to walk away, but still would have opportunity to come back. In less than a week, he called to confirm his appointment time and then came in. His manner remained reserved, but there was now a tentative involvement. He was hopeful that he would be able to lift his symptoms, but wary of the pain the process might cause.

After the initial interchange, which made me fairly certain I was working with a schizoid personality disorder (he distanced as a defense; responded to interpretations of the schizoid dilemma), the patient entered into a period of cautiously getting acquainted.

For the next several months, he spoke somewhat repetitiously of his daily life, and avoided talking about the break-in. I got accustomed to hearing about his freelance computer work, and his hopes of finding a girl-friend who would be a real partner and share his interests . . . His was an isolated, self-sufficient existence, illuminated by a few long-term acquaintances and his dedication to his computer. From time to time, I would interpret his need to feel safer by staying at a distance from the topic of the break-in. I would also interpret his dilemma—the wish to get better, while at the same time keeping open an avenue of retreat from a painful topic. Occasionally, he would start to talk about the break-in, then would come late for the next session, or miss it altogether. Each time he did this, I would point out his tendency to distance physically instead of putting his dilemma into words, as well as to perceive words as something risky that sometimes required some backing off from. Eventually, he said that the persistence of his symptoms was interfering too much with his life, and decided he would follow my implications and take more of a risk with words. I told him he would need to review his experience minutely, which would lead to discomfort, but was the pathway toward relief of symptoms. At length, after this necessary segment of character work (which strengthened the containment gradually being created by the relationship) he made up his mind, and decided to proceed with the trauma work.

I encouraged him to review explicitly what had happened that night. He was reluctant, and I appealed to his intellectual defenses once more, saying that the resolution of his symptoms was in the details he would recollect. I tried to keep a balance between the supportive statements that would speak to his traumatic anxiety (and would help him to stay closer to the work) and reassurances that he should feel free to make his own choices about pacing (which would relieve some of the pressure caused by the schizoid dilemma). He responded by taking on the task in a serious, workmanlike way.

He described minutely how he had been focused on his computer when he heard the window being raised. He told of the shock he felt when he saw the gun; the suspense of being threatened and backed toward the closet. Even when he spoke of being struck in the head by the pistol, his narrative remained detached and objective. However, I noticed he began to tap his foot, and looked briefly to the side as he talked about the closet. He hesitated then, and he questioned continuing. I reassured him that the hardest places often were the most rewarding to get through. (While doing the trauma work, I openly encouraged him, whereas I would have stepped back while doing character work alone.)

Mr. Z hesitantly began to describe partly losing consciousness in the closet. He began to perspire and wiped his forehead. Then he doggedly continued, although he was clearly experiencing increasing distress.

Pt: There's something about being closed in the closet . . . I'm not feeling too well.

Th: Try to keep going.

Pt: Are the lights dimmer? [Apparently slipping into an altered state]

Th: You may be remembering being there. Try to stay with it.

Pt: I feel dizzy, sick. It's getting darker. What's the matter with me?

Th: You're remembering as if then were now. You feel as if you're in two present times. It's O.K. Just hold onto my voice and you'll be oriented. Just try to keep remembering.

Pt: It's so dark in there. [He protectively dissociates to an observer stance in order to continue] I see myself in the corner of a dark closet. Small in the corner. I hurt. Who will come and help me?

Th: I'm here with you in present time, where you're safe. Just keep telling me what's happening back there.

Pt: It's dark. I hurt. I can't push the door open. I want someone to help me.

Th: That's how you felt then. It was so frightening that you couldn't fully experience it back then. Now you can let it all through in words, and it will be released to become a memory. And, you know, all memories fade.

Pt: [Still preoccupied with his altered state] I keep hoping someone will come. Sometimes I try the knob; kick the door. No way out. It feels like forever. Really bad.

Th: What happens next?

Pt: They're coming. They open the door. Thank God. But I still feel all alone.

Th: Do you want to tell me more?

Pt: No. I'm back now.

Th: Then let yourself come back into the room. You've done a good job, and being locked in is starting to become a memory.

Pt: [Rubbing his eyes; looking around] what happened?

Th: You just went through what therapists call an "abreaction." You have gone through such a frightening experience—being beaten and locked in the closet—that you were overwhelmed by it at the time. You put part of the experience on hold until you felt it was safe to experience it more fully. Now you have done so, it will fall more into perspective.

Pt: This is interesting. But it's very strange. I feel exhausted, but I feel lighter. What's happening to me?

Th: You'll feel disoriented for awhile. But right now, you're integrating the process you just let happen. Just let your unconscious sort things out—it's an expert. [Clarification supports the patient's reclamation of normal orientation]

Mr. Z found his balance, and left. He arrived late for the next session, and seemed cautious as he spoke.

Pt: I have to say I feel more able to deal with the break-in. Would you call that a traumatic reaction I went through?

Th: That certainly seemed to be what it was.

Pt: I've been reading up. I was traumatized by the break-in, I relived the experience, and now I'm released from my fear. Is that right?

Th: You've done your homework. All I would add is that you've not relived your experience, you've finally *lived* it. [Schizoid patients often pursue understanding of their sessions through reading and research outside the sessions. I do not discourage this as long as the pursuit is integrated in the sessions themselves. Similarly, such research seems definitely helpful for trauma sufferers—again, if it is integrated into the sessions]

Th: That is generally what happens.

Mr. Z continued to rework his experience during the next few sessions. His immediate relief gave way to night fears, which in turn gave way to some liberation from his anxieties about his apartment. One thing mainly bothered him. After the break-in, he had kicked the closet door open. In the abreaction, the door had been opened by others. Did this discredit his experience? I replied that sure signs of progress were the abatement of his symptoms. I also wondered if the memory might have been mixed with another unfinished memory. Did he recall any similar experience?

Mr. Z said that he would rather not talk about it, but during his childhood he had been locked in the closet as a punishment—something he found very disturbing. But no doubt, he said, his parents had had a good reason for using this method of discipline. He fell silent.

After a long pause, I decided to let the subject rest until he decided to reintroduce it. He was silent for much of the remaining session, and left in a quiet and thoughtful mood.

The next session, he wondered whether he should continue. I asked him whether he had met the goals he had wanted to achieve. He said that much of his fear had abated—he came and went freely from his apartment—and his nightmares had eased significantly. He said that he had found therapy an interesting process, and might be willing to return to it if other problems came up. However, he thought that he would call a halt for now, rather than extend the process into the past. After all, where would it all stop? I conceded he had done well, and agreed to his stopping of therapy, with the understanding he would return if he thought it might be helpful.

3.4.1.3. Long-term Treatment

Mr. Z returned after six months. He had had an exacerbation of his symptoms. When we explored the situation, the only notable change in his life was the presence of a significant correspondence with a female friend. Realizing that closeness was an issue for Mr. Z, I hypothesized that the new relationship might be acting as a cue for old fears. I suggested he return to puzzle things out.

Mr. Z's first experience in therapy, because of its traumatic, crisis nature, had moved at an unusually quick pace for a schizoid personality (and was probably a cause for the six-month hiatus). His second experience, focused at least in part on relationship, moved with a more characteristic slowness. My early interventions, directed to his personality disorder, had been useful for working *with* the disorder, rather than resolving it. His responses too had been given under the pressure of traumatic material more than emerging from a therapeutic relationship, which had yet to be established. It would take us three years to accomplish the more trusting phase of treatment.

For another six months he proceeded with care—not wishing to tell me too much about himself, nor wanting to evoke an unexpected abreaction, as had happened before.

I assured him: "Slowly will get you there more steadily. The process was so new to you before, you want to feel safe from any more surprises; so going gradually will help you stay with it."

As time went on, he introduced me to his daily routines (eventually I knew them by heart in detail). He began his days punctually at seven a.m.; took a long, hot shower and shave to ease the effects of often troubled sleep the night before. He brought in the paper and scanned it over coffee with milk, then tomato juice and oatmeal. Lately, he read the paper to distract his mind as much as for information. Sometimes he had an extra half-tranquilizer with his breakfast to help him into a constructive waking state with less anxiety. He organized his plans for the day, checking his appointment book for freelance business meetings and tutoring engagements. Once he had planned his day, he pulled up the covers on his bed and laid out that day's wardrobe. His clothes were kept neatly clean and pressed and, as he preferred, were all of the same subdued, monochrome effect. Once he was dressed, his anxiety began to rise if he had to leave the apartment. Sometimes, he allowed extra time to boot up his computer and do a little research; this helped him to feel more self-sufficient and calmer in his own world. Unless he had a coveted day when he did all his work at home, he would gather his nerve and move quickly out the door and straight to the subway. The day would pass busily until he faced the transition back home—the hardest one. He would begin to shake when he tried to put the key in the lock. Once in, he left the door temporarily open behind him. He had set the lights on a timer, so the apartment would already be illuminated. He would force himself to check the lock on the fire-escape grate, and then methodically examine the bedroom, bathroom, and kitchenette.

After he was rationally convinced he was alone (although he felt otherwise), he removed his coat and checked his computer for e-mail. The thought that he might have some mail was a thing that encouraged him to get through the door on the way in. If he had mail, he answered it immediately. If there was no mail, he sent some out, or engaged in more research. Soon, he relaxed enough to fix a simple meal and listen to the news. Then he returned to his computer. Around eleven o'clock, he took his tranquilizer and anti-depressant and went to bed—with a night light on, and with hopes of not having more nightmares about vague, dark, threatening places. Often he was too apprehensive to fall asleep, and kept the television on in the background. He would fitfully doze in and out of late shows and late movies, until a steadier sleep finally came.

By seven a.m. the daily routine began again.

The sessions were interrupted by silences, so that some time elapsed before Mr. Z's routine was clear to me. After that, I slowly began to learn about his work life (he didn't like to be told what to do); and his e-mail acquaintances, who were primarily interested in computers, chess, and science fiction. Eventually, he began to talk about Claudia, an e-mail correspondent and science fiction fan. They had once worked in the same office, and shared conversations over Aazimov's *Foundation* series of novels. When he left the office (he didn't think his boss appreciated his work), they continued to correspond by computer. Although they were both single and enjoyed many subjects in common, they did not meet in person after Mr. Z left the job. Mr.

Z thought he would like to see Claudia again, but worried that she would want to go dancing. He had tried dancing lessons, but lost patience with the instructor.

I noted that his life seemed to be limited by his reluctance to work with an authority figure. He answered that he was aware of this, but sensed much irritation in giving over control to another person. He didn't think he was likely to change.

I wondered whether he might not have lunch with Claudia, as he sometimes did with his male correspondents. He said he had been thinking of this, but lunch might lead to supper, and then to dancing and so he hesitated. And no, it wasn't the thought of a sexual encounter that stopped him. He had had several brief liaisons, and thought sex wouldn't be a problem.

I asked: "Why not go to lunch with her, anyway? You've both been talking about it for several months. If she wants to take it further, why can't you tell her about your concern?" He said it was easier not to bring up a problematic subject. I replied: "But this is a puzzle you should consider solving for yourself! You're only using one way of handling a problematic situation—by distancing from it. Think of all the ways you have of getting out of a spot on your computer! You can hit "escape," or "un-do," or maybe exit the program. Maybe there are other things you can do, too, depending on your expertise. In this case, the only alternative you're choosing is to distance yourself by giving up the computer." He thought for a long time. Then: "You're saying I could use words and strategy to modify a situation. Then I might have something instead of nothing."

After a couple of weeks, Mr. Z invited Claudia to lunch, and she accepted without mentioning either dinner or dancing.

After this hopeful beginning, Mr. Z resumed his customary routine for a period of time. I returned to my usual slow motion attention, reminding myself that working with a schizoid personality meant a wary progression like a walk over thin ice. It was difficult not to let my mind wander, grow impatient, or resign myself to the countertransferential role of subservience, controlled by his rigidity.

One day I noticed I was unusually restless, and realized 1) I was letting myself become more passive and watching the clock frequently; 2) his range of information was shrinking, and he hadn't mentioned Claudia for awhile.

I brought to his attention that he was saying less and that the sessions seemed to be less communicative—I wondered if he might be drawing back for some reason. He thought, then said insightfully: "Ever since I had lunch with Claudia I've been feeling closed in. I suppose I should have talked about it with her. But I was afraid I'd hurt her feelings, so I just stopped asking her out." "And you didn't mention it in here, either." Another silence—a longer one—then he asked: "Why would I feel crowded by you?" "Perhaps it's because it's about your private life, and that feels too close to home." Silence.

Pt: Are you saying the more used I get to someone, the more I want to get away?"

Th: Close. I'm saying the more you get used to someone, the more feelings you have about them, and the more you want to get away from those feelings.

Pt: Why should feelings of closeness make me want to distance?

Th: The only way to find that out is to stay with the feelings, and keep talking about them.

Pt: [Long silence] I'm going to think this over. Can I call you in a month and let you know if I decide to continue?

We discussed this awhile, with my pointing out that he was showing exactly the behavior we had been discussing. Asking him to keep in mind this reaction to discussing subjects close to home, I agreed to the hiatus.

After a month, he came back again. He clearly had been taking the time to think, and had used his intellectual defenses well.

Pt: It's a lot about patterns, isn't it?

Th: Could you explain more?

Pt: The more I make a relationship work, the more I want to get away from it. Is that something I'm supposed to be learning here?

Th: Yes. It's a paradoxical pattern we've observed—you take a step forward, get uncomfortable feelings, and want to take a step back again.

Pt: And the more I want to understand these feelings, the more I have to stay put and experience them.

Th: Yes.

Pt: I think I found another pattern, too. [Silence] Staying away from Claudia and from therapy made me feel in outer space. Sort of empty. Kind of a reverse running away from my feelings—if I get too far away. I get bad feelings, too.

Th: If you get too close, you become apprehensive, but too much distance makes you uncomfortable, too.

Pt: My reactions to my apartment are getting worse, too. [Silence] I guess the only way is to go straight ahead, no matter how I feel.

Th: And to talk it through to understanding.

[Silence]

Th: Is it possible that you felt frustrated because I didn't help you more with your symptoms?

Pt: [Hesitantly] Yes. And I never talked to you about that, either. [Pause] I never mentioned how I didn't want to talk about my symptoms, either. That time I went through that experience—that "abreaction"—gave me such horrible feelings I didn't want to chance it again. But I don't think it's over.

Th: Why is that?

Pt: I think there's more in my childhood. The closet. I don't feel ready to go back there, although I think I have to.

Th: So it sounds you need to feel more secure in present time. Otherwise, you'll feel that strong pull to go away again.

Pt: Yes. I need to find a way to feel safer.

Mr. Z's intellectual defenses were carrying him forward. I hoped that the increasing therapeutic relationship was also supporting the process. An encouraging sign was his willingness to allow himself negative feelings toward me.

Pt: You know, I've felt you were like my mother, overseeing every detail of my life. When I drink tomato juice in the morning, I say 'Dr. O knows I'm drinking this.' So I changed what I'm drinking—I won't tell you what to—and now I feel better.

Th: Maybe the time has come to talk more about your parents.

Pt: I think you're right—my patterns go back to there—but I feel very uncomfortable.

Th: So once more you find yourself with one foot outside the door and the other foot in. The choice is yours, whichever way you decide to step.

He began to talk more about his childhood—talking almost as much about how uncomfortable this made him. But he stayed with it.

His father was a rigid perfectionist, who expected the patient to know how to act mature at five years old. No matter how much the patient struggled to fulfil his role, he was still a child. So his father beat him mercilessly with a belt (the buckle end), and locked him in the closet. The times in the closet were very long. The patient grew hungry, was forced to urinate in the corner (which brought on later beatings), and called for his mother until he realized he would not be answered. This treatment continued until his pre-teens, when he was able to respond more like the adult his father wanted him to be. But before that time, the hours in the closet took on a life of their own. The isolation frightened and dismayed him, and then became a unique experience. The hunger and loneliness were joined by shooting colors and strange bodily sensations. He felt as though he were disappearing. When they let him out of the closet, he would be stunned and unable to react.

Pt: How could I have been so bad as to deserve this?

Th: If you saw this happening to another child, would you say the child was bad? Wouldn't you feel for the child? [Cognitive]

Pt: I feel bad because they made me feel bad. Oh God, how do I free myself from this feeling?

We were cautiously approaching his feelings, guided by his clear and insightful intelligence. I asked him: "Now that you're in touch with the bad feelings your parents gave you, are you willing to stay with your past recollections and take hold in present time?"

After a long pause, he replied: "I can't run away. It will just go with me. But this is very hard. My parents were the only ones there for me. How can I think badly of them?"

I replied: "You know, all human beings are a mixture of things, and so were your parents. They protected you, but they also hurt you. Perhaps your father felt he had to discipline you like that because of how he was disciplined as a child. Perhaps your mother went along because she was always told to support her husband."

He did not reply. He was silent until the end of the session. When he returned, he had been thinking things through for himself again.

He said: "The closet, the darkness represent my parents' cruelty. They meant well, I think, but still they were cruel. My whole life has become that dark closet. If I stay in it, I'll fall through the bottom of the world. If I come out, I'll be beaten again. I think I sometimes see the closet as refuge—at least I'm alone with my thoughts, and no one will beat me there. But I'm losing myself in there. There's no safe way."

A long silence passed.

Pt: Is it all right to think this way?

Th: Of course. You are using your good common sense to help you stay with difficult and deeply conflicted feelings.

He pursued this theme for several weeks, during which time he admitted wanting to run away, but also said he was determined to transcend his dilemma. "I need to separate the present from the past," he said. "They locked me up in the closet then, but now I'm free to walk out on my own." This insightful patient took his resolution a step further. "I'm setting myself free from the closet, but I'm also setting my parents free from the blame of putting me there. The closet is the past; my father is gone and my mother probably doesn't remember. I'm the only one who can shut myself in the closet now, and it's time I stopped. No more closets." We reviewed in detail his being locked in the closet, but he did not repeat the initial abreaction that had linked present to past. He was more willing to admit and stay with his feelings, but these seemed more distant now.

Mr. Z continued to stay and do the work. He was pleased with his progress, and liked to conceptualize it as he went along. Alongside our work together, he seemed to be doing a parallel process of therapy, using his intellect and capacity for observation. I began to suspect he also was doing independent reading to satisfy his need for a sense of control. The independent research was evident in his occasional (correct) usage of such terms as "individuation," "maladaptive defenses," and "real self." When I asked him about this, he said he liked to support his experience with theoretical data.

He surprised me once with the following statement: "I think I'm no longer relating to you by transference acting out. I'm staying and talking to you about my uncertainties instead of putting my fears into behavior and running away. I suppose you could now say we have a classic transference relationship—I see you more as yourself, but sometimes I feel you crowd me like my mother. But I've noticed the more I talk about things, the more like yourself you seem and the realer I feel. I would guess we have a therapeutic alliance."

I was almost too startled to validate him. Then I asked whether I glimpsed a sense of humor behind all this data. He gave a small smile, and said his "inner child" could sometimes be "an imp."

The abused child in him was beginning to play.

One day he told me that he had invited Claudia for supper. I did not press him further, and he eventually followed up with an astonishing piece of information.

Unable to tolerate a teacher, he had ordered a number of discs on dance instruction for his computer. In time, he invited Claudia to a supper dance, and there discovered that he had taught himself well. They were both pleased, and agreed to go dancing again.

I do not know how the relationship turned out. I only know that my patient was pleased with his new freedom to assert himself, and that he was insistent on forgiving his past. Did anger remain? I think so. Will he return to treatment for further working through? It is possible. But I do know he had made a deeper peace with himself and his inner world, while also acknowledging that scars go deep, and healing is rarely complete. However, as he made reference to his childhood abuse, his symptoms abated significantly—not only did he not abreact, but the tension of the telling no longer brought him anxiety; his dreams were rarely disturbed, and he came and went from) his apartment freely. He knew that we are able to resolve much, but may need future opportunities to resolve more. His quick mind helped him to know that sometimes we intellectually grasp more that we are able to match emotionally, but that the gap can be steadily narrowed, given the will to persist.

CHAPTER 4

SPECIAL ISSUES

4.1. The Challenge of Dissociative Identity Disorder (MPD)

(Note: DID is listed in DSM-IV as a dissociative disorder, not as a personality disorder. However, extensive clinical experience leads me to believe that the host—or presenting—personality invariably carries a personality disorder. The alternative—or split-off—personalities defensively carry the traumatic experiences. The balancing of character work and trauma work becomes very concrete in DID, as the strengthening of the host personality is measured against the gradual release of traumatic experience from the alters. The therapeutic goal is the eventual acceptance into consciousness of the traumatic history by the host personality, thereby eliminating the need for dissociative alters.)

Of all the pathological results of early trauma, probably DID (dissociative identity disorder) is one of the most severe and controversial outcomes. DID (also known as MPD—multiple personality disorder), as an alternative to madness and death, is an impressive defense, but one that engenders confusion, curiosity and even skepticism in the therapeutic community as well as the general society.

Among those who specialize in work with this disorder, there is agreement that DID arises from early, consistent, unabating, extreme abuse (Kluft, 1988, p. 212). The intensity of the abuse leads to splitting-off of parts of the self that hold pain, so that the primary self can continue to function under conditions that would be overwhelming for a conscious, integrated self to bear.

DSM-IV (1994, p. 484) reports that DID "reflects a failure to integrate various aspects of identity, memory, and consciousness. Each personality state may be experienced as if it has a distinct personal history, self-image, and identity, including a separate name." There must be two or more of these personality states, each "with its own relatively enduring pattern of perceiving, relating to, and thinking about the environment and self" (p. 487). Further, "at least two of these identities . . . recurrently take control of the person's behavior" (p. 487).

In the 1970's and 80's, interest in DID led to exciting exploration and theory-forming. Dissention both inside and outside the field of psychotherapy, plus the unhappy involvement of the courts, have lately transformed theoretical speculation into legal risk-taking. Since multiples and others who have been abused early on have been taking their grievances to court; parents have been striking back. A moral issue has become a situation in which a parent goes to court and a therapist loses a license. Intimidation has become the focus, where healing was to be the goal. As a result, the patients suffer, as therapists draw away from their cases out of a sense of self-preservation.

I believe my patients (since I do not choose to work with patients I cannot believe). But I tell them that court procedures are not a part of therapy. The need to heal the self must be satisfied, and tribunals are not a form of resolution within.

Let us return to the clinical phenomenon.

4.1.1. The structure of multiplicity

The multiple characteristically puts forward a "host" personality, that is a presenting, or executive personality, to introduce the self. The host personality carries on daily activities and relationships, more or less like a non-multiple. But the host may experience gaps in time, or may appear to introduce her/himself under a different name with different mannerisms, and not be aware of it. The presence of an "alter" (or alternative personality)—or more than one—can be deduced from this. Another sub-self has temporarily taken over the functioning of the body.

It appears that the primary self has fragmented over years of abuse, and that the partial selves have cohered around specific ego states and experiences (Putnam, 1989, p. 54). These dissociated selves are of two primary types: (1) They have been divided off to protect the essential self from experiencing (fully remembering) traumatic states; (2) They have been divided off to preserve ego strengths that might have been crushed if consciousness had remained complete.

Unfortunately, those alters who protect from knowledge of trauma are often identified with the victim or the aggressor, while the exclusion of ego strengths from the host personality increases the tendency to give way to victimized or aggressive states. We are looking at a self that has all the ingredients to know and synthesize itself, except that the defensive barriers of dissociation prevent self-knowledge, and the host personality is afraid to relinquish those barriers.

Why does the host personality put up such barriers? The host carries a personality disorder that resists knowledge of the past, which brings loss of idealized relationship, and assault by devastating feelings. The pain of abandonment depression and the impact of delayed trauma threaten to catch the self in an unbearable vise.

Anyone who has worked with or read about multiples knows that the alters carry a variety of psychic states: personality disorders (including sociopathy), psychosis, and even states that seem quite normal. Why should the host carry a predominating personality disorder? I speculate that, if a human being is not to come apart completely, there must be some governing structure to the psyche. We are familiar with the pathology of personality disorder, but perhaps have not given it its due as a defense against psychic annihilation. It may stand as the last barricade against loss of reality or life because it is a tough (though rigid) structure that has dissociation as a last, powerful weapon. A part of the self must be given up to preserve the presenting self, although the result will be depletion.

Arguments are made for the disregarding of alters as a manipulative fabrication rather than a life saving defense. For example, the Guidelines *(1999)* for treating DID, issued by the International Society for the Study of Dissociation, warns the practitioner against encouraging the patient to "create" new alters during the therapy process. In my experience, alters rarely appear who are not part of the defense against past trauma (at the time the trauma occurred), or as part of the self system intended to preserve ego strength as old traumatic issues emerge (a prelude to the conscious self's assuming this task).

I believe that the alters are always a defensive part of that elusive phenomenon we call the self, and must be fully acknowledged and allowed to realize themselves in the therapeutic process.

The overcoming of identity discontinuity can only be repaired by encouraging realization of the alters who represent gaps in consciousness. This co-consciousness cannot be achieved without the alters identifying themselves to the therapist, to each other, and to the host personality. Integration follows naturally as the core self accepts disowned parts of the self—essentially as it happens in a less-vivid disorder, where divided-off parts of the self are not personified. We acknowledge ourselves fully in order to accept who we are.

I recall working with a patient whose child alter told me the story of her abuse, then seemed to fall asleep while reciting a favorite story. I found that she had integrated. "But why?" I asked, "What made it possible?" The answer was "because she has been acknowledged enough." This was my first realization that integration is not a matter of coercion or dismissal of alters. Integration is the recognition of divided-off parts of the self, their stories and their issues, until they feel free to blend with the host, and the host feels safe enough to take them back.

The "front" is the name I use for the primary alters. There tend to be about a dozen or fewer of them, and they may be the only representatives of the inner world, or may intervene on behalf of others. They usually present themselves as a non-group, especially since they may stand for opposing characteristics: aggression, concern, studiousness, flirtatiousness, etc. I find it crucial to know each individually, and to encourage them to form an executive committee. I find I am most listened to if I emphasize the safety of the body and the protection of the child alters (of which there may be many, with only one or two representatives on this level). When the front pools its resources, it is effective, since the individuals complement each other. There usually is a helper in the front, who can advise as to the nature of the multiple system and to the direction and pacing of the therapy.

An initial challenge is to assist the host in recognizing the front—a process that may take as long as the therapy itself. One of the protective features of DID dissociation is that the host knows nothing of the insiders, and so cannot give their presence away.

What happens when the host becomes aware of the insiders? Since this marks an important relinquishment of defense, it is resisted. Even after the multiple systems have been accepted, the host will go into denial. It is a shaky bridge to cross.

The alters are relatively clear about their roles, but the host personality resists acknowledging them as a simple personality disorder would resist knowing abusive memories and letting go maladaptive defenses for self-supporting inner strengths. The double task here is for the executive personality to accept not only the qualities contained by the alters, but to allow expansion of self-boundaries that will permit the reclamations of divided-off parts of the self.

4.1.2. The clinical approach to multiplicity

Except in those cases where the front presents itself immediately (or even in place of the host personality), DID should, at first, be approached as any other personality disorder. The host's personality should be diagnosed and treated accordingly, in order to provide as secure a containment as possible for the whole self. While the host maintains a pronounced personality disorder, it will use the typical maladaptive defenses of personality disorder to manage additional stresses of feeling or memory. When understanding begins to supplant acting out, denial, projection, etc., and the therapeutic alliance is forming, it is safest for the therapy to include work with the front.

It has been a common experience of mine that some patients will not reveal their multiplicity (which may or may not have been hypothesized by the therapist) until this first stage of containment is somewhat in place. I have written elsewhere (1995, p. 235) about my first DID patient, who had done extensive character work before undergoing a period of confusion and dissociation that led to the emergence of the front.

There often seems to be a self-protectiveness in the multiple that does not permit an unfolding of the inner world unless there is a certain psychic preparedness in the host personality. This is a major reason why the therapist should not press for a diagnosis of DID before it becomes a logical outcome of the work (the simplest, and probably most frequent show of this preparedness is the appearance of an alter—or alters—who supplants the host personality to introduce her/himself). The therapy then becomes a juggling act more complicated than therapy with the usual personality disorder.

The therapist continues to strengthen the patient's system by conventional character and trauma work with the host personality. This means strengthening defenses and the capacity for self-observation in order to tolerate the personality disorder defenses that guard against feelings of abandonment depression.

- The therapist takes time to meet with and understand the members of the front. The therapist's capacity to understand the alters, encourage their intercooperation, and tolerate their abuse histories, prefigures the host personality's ability to eventually contain the whole system, its diversity and its pain. (If the front has already emerged at the beginning of treatment, the alters should be acknowledged. The task of encouraging them to support each other and the host personality must begin at this point, with every effort taken to enlist the front to ally with the host's character work.)

- The therapist facilitates communication between the host and the alters, preparing the ground for this becoming a spontaneous happening.

- During steps 2) and 3), the therapist must be careful not to let too much information come into conscious expression too quickly. Traumatic material must always be weighed against the capacity of the host to absorb it. This material should be maximally contained when the host is coping with such powerful feelings as abandonment depression.

- Periods of consolidation should be allowed for a system that is balancing and pacing the absorption of near-intolerable quantities and types of material.

- If additional alters emerge behind the front, they will tend to group according to age, type of abuse experienced (or perpetrated), or abusive episode. They also will fall into categories of victim, perpetrator, protector, and helper. The therapy may sometimes be shortened when the alters are addressed as one of these groupings. (I have described the inner world of the highly complex multiple in detail elsewhere [Orcutt, 1995, pp. 237-252].)

- Integration is not always the goal for patients. In that case, the goals become co-consciousness and intercooperation, so that the person functions with continuity of the self, and with minimal conflict.
- The judicial use of hypnosis is valuable for therapy with these patients, who spend so much of their being in a trance state. Hypnosis should be used to facilitate, not to lead: to help ease the telling of abuse, and to foster a sense of calm and safety. Informed consent, of course, must be given.

Therapy of DID thus becomes a multi-juggling act for the therapist, who must balance character work with both host personality and alters, do trauma work with all personalities, and synthesize the work, as well, to achieve new levels of self-integration. When integration can be taken to its fullest, the result is the reclamation of a whole self.

4.2. The "Sliding Diagnosis"

My experience with what I have termed the "sliding diagnosis," is not found in the literature. Over and over, students and supervisees have presented me with the same problem. The patient's diagnosis will not stay put. Borderlines balk at confrontation, and need mirroring interpretation; narcissists unpredictably respond only to interpretations of the schizoid dilemma. These patients often had an abuse history in common, or symptoms and behavior that suggested such a background.

Two possibilities would have to be considered. First, an outright misdiagnosis. Second, the chance that traumatic material may have been emerging, which would require a shift in intervention to the more directly supportive. But, after misdiagnoses have been ruled out, and after cognitive interventions have been introduced to manage intrusions of traumatic reactions into the character pattern, the diagnosis may still seem to slide around.

Can a patient have more than one personality disorder? Even the multiple personality disorder, whose self is fragmented into sub-selves with varying diagnoses, maintains an executive (host) personality with a focal personality disorder. It appears that a basic cohesiveness of the self is reliant on maintaining a primary focus of conflict: a predominating diagnosis.

What hypothesis can be used to guide the treatment of these patients? The answer seems to lie in the picture of early abuse that arises in many of these cases. During the formative years, the patient has been subjected to severe mistreatment, and so may regress to deeply entrenched secondary fixation points that exert an influence close to that of the primary fixation point. It is the constancy of the abuse over the formative years, the vulnerability of the child over that period, or probably a combination of both in the caregiver-child relationship that creates the tendency of the diagnosis to "slide."

It seems that there has been so much duress over the formative years, that each phase of development has been a candidate for primary developmental arrest until the decisive damage was done.

The points of secondary fixation have been so close in intensity to the primary point, that excessive stress could cause a temporary slippage back to the earlier, secondary place of psychic arrest.

Juggling all these interventions at once presents yet another challenge for the therapist working with the personality disordered patient who also suffers from psychic trauma. The work requires close listening for shifts in the patient's response, especially when the session topics grow more stressful. Listening to the patient's reactions to interventions is also a guide. The therapist must keep in mind, however, that the patient will eventually revert to the primary diagnosis, and the basic intervention must be returned to.

Case example: Linda Q has been diagnosed as having borderline personality disorder. Typical interchanges run as follows:

Pt: My boss called me into the office to discuss my lateness. I felt so angry. I can never do anything right. I'm just no good.

Th: Your boss wanted to guide you to improve your work habits. Why wouldn't you want to use this to your advantage? [Confrontation.]

Pt: He makes me feel like a bad little child.

Th: No . . . you make yourself feel this way. If you feel his criticism is an attack, why do you have to join him? Why not stay on your own side and use the information to your benefit?

[Confrontation.]

Pt: I guess I just get too hard on myself. [Integrating the confrontation.]

Then the patient departs from the usual pattern of responses, and confrontation fails:

Pt: Now my boss is calling me into his office for my frequent absences. It makes me feel just awful.

Th: Why should you feel awful when he's trying to help you do your job better?

[Confrontation.]

Pt: You don't understand. It makes me feel so frightened.

Th: Why should you feel frightened of someone who's trying to help you?

[Confrontation.]

Pt: No, no. [Refusing confrontation.] You're scaring me. I'm afraid I'll lose my job, and even my therapist doesn't understand. [Under fear of loss, seems to show narcissistic vulnerability. Confrontation doesn't work. Change tack?]

Th: The fear of loss frightens you so much, that you try to protect yourself by seeking my support. [Mirroring interpretation of narcissistic vulnerability.]

Pt: That's right. It's so painful to be misunderstood. It makes me feel small and abused.

Th: So it's important to understand that, when you're criticised or disbelieved, you feel back in that place where you feel hurt instead of understood. [Cognitive acknowledgment of early abuse.]

159

Pt: (In tears.) It hurts so much to feel so small and
       helpless and hated. I know it comes from the past,
       but the pain is so much in the present. [Emotionally
       confirmed insight.]

The therapist, as in the above example, may have to shift
from confrontation to mirroring interpretation of narcissistic
vulnerability, to cognitive interpretation of reactions to
early abuse to help the patient get in touch with the deeper
feelings evoked by her job situation.

Work with the "sliding diagnosis" truly tests the "third
ear" of the therapist, as well as the therapist's skill in using
different interventions. But once the concept is mastered, it
shows the way through an otherwise confusing, potentially
dead-ended maze of defense.

The "sliding diagnosis" is a guide to treatment, and
also a guide to the refining of the patient's diagnosis. As
I have worked with my own patients, and taught the
"sliding diagnosis" to numerous experienced therapists I
have supervised, the diagnosis of persistent developmental
trauma usually has been confirmed, or at least has been
brought forward as a clear possibility.

The "sliding diagnosis" can be added to the diagnostic
signs of early overt or hidden psychic trauma, along with
acting out of sexual or violent behavior, avoidance of
sexuality, risk-taking, or excessive reliance on dissociation or
denial (including physical numbing) in sexual situations.

In the case of the patient whose early trauma was
unknown or suspected, the presence of the "sliding
diagnosis" can clarify the diagnostic picture.

4.3. The Complexity of Transference and Countertransference when Personality Disorder and Traumatic Stress are Comorbid

The issues of transference and countertransference are among the most complex in dynamic psychotherapy. The definitions have been evolving ever since Freud originated the concepts. Transference and countertransference are often subjectively perceived and elusive.

They are unconscious or preconscious, and are based on the interpersonal process, which can be objectified to some extent in observed behavior and through associations, but which remains largely emotional and subjective. The management of these issues depends to a great extent on the therapist's neutrality, empathy, intuition, and experience.

Freud (1912, pp. 312ff.) originally described transference as the patient's distortion of the analytic relationship, based on past parental conflict and projected onto the analyst in present time. Countertransference is the mirror image of transference: it is the analyst's own transference projected onto the analysand (Freud, 1910, p. 289).

Freud's definitions refer to the patient whose psyche has matured enough to project a misperception of the therapist onto a separate, whole object. As treatment has expanded to examine the "bipersonal field" (Langs, 1976), and to explore the relationship between the therapist and the "pre-Oedipal" patient (Giovacchini, 1979; Masterson, 1983; Searles, 1979; Spotnitz, 1979) the definition of transference/countertransference has widened. The transference that reflects its origins in the earliest years of life affects relationship more globally. The patient not only perceives relationship without clear discrimination between past and present, but puts that perception into action.

In other words, the patient does not see the therapist as making a critical remark, but as wholly critical. In addition, the patient does not discuss this situation as a hypothetical problem to be clarified, but reacts as if uncompromisingly criticised.

In such an instance, attempts at classical interpretation would be seen as further criticism, and reacted to accordingly.

Masterson (1983) examines the nature of the pre-Oedipal transference, which he calls "transference acting-out," and its countertransferential impact on the therapist:

> . . . the patient's "business" or objective in the session is to evoke countertransference reactions that enable him/her to avoid the intrapsychic nature of the conflict. The emotions themselves are so primitive and powerful . . . that they can suddenly provoke the therapist to respond and catch him or her in the patient's acting out trap. (p. 296)

Masterson continues, describing how the patient's transference acting out pulls the therapist toward a distortion of the therapeutic process:

> . . . the patient leads with his transference acting-out, and the therapist follows with his countertransference. This catapults the therapist into an intrapsychic struggle of his/her own to identify countertransference and regain a therapeutically objective perspective. (p. 296)

If the therapist is successful in holding a neutral stance, the therapeutic process continues:

> . . . [The therapist] takes over and leads the patient by confronting [in the case of the borderline] the transference acting-out. This sends the patient back into an intrapsychic investigation to understand his conflicts, which in turn triggers intense affect in the patient, which may then again evoke a countertransference in the therapist. (p. 296)

The goal of understanding transference with the (pre-Oedipal) personality disorder is twofold. The first goal is to maintain therapeutic neutrality. The second goal is to help the patient transform acting out into insight and eventually to change transference acting-out into classical transference within a therapeutic alliance.

What is the difference between a relationship dominated by transference acting-out and the working relationship called the therapeutic alliance? How is this situation complicated by psychic trauma?

As Freud pointed out (1914) and Masterson reiterates (1981, 146 ff.), the repetition compulsion rules acting out. The patient who is transferentially acting-out is repeating an aspect of childhood relationship disturbing to face by direct understanding. The patient is repeating unawares the dysfunctional way in which he or she was shaped in the formative years.

These formative years were dyadic, and in order for the transference acting-out to be complete, the patient seeks to shape the therapist (or spouse, or lover, friend, or child) into a complementary form that will repeat the early scenario. The patient tries to recreate the original parent-child misattunement that, in the early years, set the scene for personality disorder. Paradoxical though it may seem, through early interpersonal programming and later defense, the patient repeats the interaction rather than the underlying feeling, and is caught in an endless behavioral trap. The therapist may be caught in a corresponding countertransference acting-out trap, in which case the early damage will become more entrenched.

As I once described this:

> In their simplest form, inductions from the patient tend to shape us to the role of the early partner. The way we find ourselves unthinkingly responding to the patient tends to recapitulate the mother of the borderline, who encourages compliance or gets into a power struggle; or the narcissistic mother, who requires her child be an extension of herself, or the mother of the schizoid, who hardly experiences her child as more than a function. (Orcutt, 1996, p. 208)

The patient defensively draws the therapist into a recreation of the original dyadic malfunction. The clinging or oppositional borderline evokes falsely rewarding or angrily withdrawing behavior from the therapist.

The therapist may be intimidated into an admiring oneness with the manifest narcissist, or may constantly push and nag the hesitant, over-responsible closet narcissist toward assertive action. Or the effect of the schizoid's slow caution may evoke an annoyance which leads the therapist to treat the patient unempathically.

The therapist may be aware of being shaped into a role complementary to the patient's disorder, in which case the therapist may monitor him or herself as a guide to maintaining neutrality, clarifying diagnosis, and intervening appropriately. Properly monitored, the patient's attempt to shape the therapist's response into a repetition of the original dyadic misattunement offers a unique window into the patient's past.

How is this phenomenon accomplished? When the patient is manifestly acting out (the borderline may be self-mutilating; the narcissist may be blatantly self-absorbed; the schizoid may be interminably "untouchable") the therapist's reactions are pulled toward becoming the response of an untrained layman, and are easily identified. But there is usually a more subtle level of influence, which increases with the relationship between patient and therapist, and may affect the most sophisticated professional.

The defense most closely identified with countertransference and countertransference acting-out is projective identification. Allan Schore (1999) has pioneered in the psychoneurological exploration of this phenomenon, which may be as much a primitive means of communication as a defense. Shore describes projective identification as non-verbal, right frontal lobe activity that causes a synchrony between mother and child because of their unique closeness, and because of the necessity for the mother to act as psychic regulator for the emotionally vulnerable child. The biological mechanism is not understood, but there is evidence for the mother's "intuitive" reception of her child's feelings, and a similar happening appears to take place between the therapist and the pre-Oedipal patient.

How does this present in the clinical situation? The therapist becomes aware of an intense feeling—often anger, but it may be sorrow, relief, or any other feeling—that could easily be mistaken for the therapist's own.

Therapists are probably most familiar with sudden, inexplicable feelings of anger or helplessness, but projective identification can evoke feelings of joy, disgust, attraction, terror, sadness, and so on. (Orcutt, 1996, p. 207)

If the therapist is familiar with the phenomenon, projective identification will be experienced as an intrusion into the flow of the therapist's neutrality, and will need to be observed before commented upon. Even if the feeling is only held (without verbal comment) the therapist has made an important non-verbal intervention: the therapist has absorbed the patient's overflow of feeling without acting out countertransferentially. (The importance of the therapist's neutral stance can be further explored. Far from being cold and passive, this is an emotionally-containing, positive position the therapist takes actively on behalf of a continued healthy therapeutic relationship. Here, Winnicott's concept of the "holding environment" comes to mind [1960, pp. 43-44].)

How is this dealt with in the clinical situation? It cannot be stressed enough that the first step is one of forbearance and self-examination on the part of the therapist. Typically, the patient who is using projective identification is placing in the therapist feelings not yet fully tolerable in the self. For instance, when the patient "puts" unacceptable anger into the therapist if the therapist reacts with unexpected anger, the result is a repetition of the mother's inability to "hold" the distress of her young child. Countertransference acting-out has taken place, and the patient once more feels victimized and inadequate. However, if the therapist remains focused and calm, and simply remarks on a certain sense of tension in the room, this may help the patient to reclaim pre-processed feeling and begin to deal with it subjectively.

The inductions from patient to therapist to act out countertransferentially are strong and subtle, and need more scientific understanding. For now, we can recognize them and use the information they give us, rather than fall into the dyadic repetition compulsion that is the special pitfall of work with personality disorder.

The repetition compulsion also rules over the maladaptive management of physical/sexual trauma experienced in the formative years. Developmental trauma, like the mechanism that creates personality disorder, appears to be "remembered" non-verbally in the right hemisphere, and cannot find its way into words and resolution through an interaction with the left hemisphere. Only the therapeutic relationship can evoke, hold, and work through the old experience to find a new way of being in release of feeling and conscious verbalization.

What are the implications for the simultaneous presence of personality disorder and developmental trauma? When these states are comorbid, transference and countertransference acting-out have a potential for being intensified.

First, consider the most common dyadic possibilities of developmental trauma:

Victim	↔	Abuser
Abuser	↔	Victim
Victim	↔	Rescuer
Victim	↔	Observer

The abused person may act out his history by being re-abused or turning victimizer. He might also take the role of rescuer or observer. The patient may also attempt to mould the therapist into a complementary type, especially if the predisposition is already set by the therapist's own background (how many are drawn to the therapeutic role because of an initial need to rescue?)

The reader already may have noticed that the personality disorder dyads and the trauma dyads may be similar. Following are some of the possibilities:

Victim borderline	↔	Abusive therapist
Abusive borderline	↔	Victim therapist
Victim borderline	↔	Rescuing therapist
Abusive narcissist	↔	Victim *I* abusive therapist
Idealizing victim narcissist	↔	Rescuing therapist
Distant victim schizoid	↔	Observing therapist

These are only some of the more typical permutations of the therapeutic misalliance. The point here is twofold. 1) The personality disorder must be resolved sufficiently to allow it to be separated from the trauma work. 2) The therapist must be especially attentive to the differentiation of the impact of the patient's behavior and projections, because they come from a comorbid origin.

Case example: I had worked many years with Annie X, a specially rambunctious borderline personality whose diagnosis had been complicated by early traumatic parental abuse. Her escapades with men, alcohol, and overdosing had tried my therapeutic neutrality, but somehow had not broken it. Annie had overcome much of her characterological acting out, but had slumped into an abandonment depression with marked passive-aggressive features. Annie was acting silent, helpless, and awful, and was in danger of losing her job—Nothing I said was of use. Confrontation left her in silence. I escalated my confrontations and then, faced with her inert helplessness, found myself rising to my feet and ordering her out of my office. Since she was disinclined to move, and only stared at me, I had time to pull myself together, sit down, and recommence acting like a therapist. At this juncture, I realized that her stubbornness and opposition had aroused feelings of violence in me, as it may have in her own parents. I took a different tack, and acknowledged that sometimes she must feel so cornered by life that there seemed to be nothing for her to do but dig in her heels.

This remark, addressed to her traumatized self, drew a response from her, and she said she felt without a guide, and unwilling to make any move in her own behalf. During this phase of therapy, I continued to simply acknowledge her helplessness and frustration, rather than confront it, and she continued to be responsive. She began to struggle to understand her interpersonal world more than she would have if I had continued to work with her personality disorder with minimal attention to the trauma. In addition, her job performance began to improve.

Once again, I had to remind myself: After we have become aware that we have been pulled in, identify the origins of our feelings in the patient's acting-out defense, and reclaim our neutral stance, we have, in effect, initiated a therapeutic process. When we weaken the patient's repetition compulsion by refusing to enact one half of the pathological dyad, we have actually begun to interrupt the patient's entire acting-out defense. (Orcutt, 1996, p. 208)

4.4. The use of hypnosis in the integration of a childhood trauma memory

As Lacan observed, the unconscious is a language, and hypnosis "speaks" that "language" by evoking the five senses and using metaphor and association. Use of hypnosis to uncover traumatic events of early childhood has become controversial; ideally, these events should be corroborated by witnesses, material evidence, or at least by the patient's dreams, associations, sensations, or repetitive symbolic behavior. In my experience, I have found the use of hypnosis catalytic in some cases where thorough character work has failed to resolve the patient's pain, and recurring symptoms suggest there may be underlying trauma.

In another situation, the patient's personality may have been strengthened to the point where the spontaneous emergence of traumatic material is tolerated, and in this instance, hypnosis may be especially useful in promoting a sense of calm and containment. In any event, trauma work using hypnosis, like any trauma work, should be supported by solid character work and (if necessary) appropriate medication.

Since I wrote the following piece, the language of psychotherapy itself has been changing. I might now refer to the "unconscious" as the "non-verbal memory system," or perhaps the "right brain:' "crossing the repression barrier" might be called "integrating the verbal and non-verbal memory systems."

A note about the patient. Seven years after the publication of this piece, Diana continues to be a highly successful corporate executive.

CHAPTER 5

UNCOVERING "FORGOTTEN" CHILD ABUSE IN PSYCHOTHERAPY OF A BORDERLINE DISORDER OF THE SELF[*]

5.1. Uncovering "Forgotten" Child Abuse in the Psychotherapy of a Borderline Disorder of the Self

At a 1990 Masterson conference, I presented an ongoing case that appeared to exemplify the Masterson Approach to the diagnosis and treatment of an upper-level borderline disorder of the self. The patient, referred to as Diana, was very bright and highly functioning. She had been intensely motivated to pursue the nearly five years of psychotherapy (increasing after two years from one to two sessions a week) that helped her to correct maladaptive defenses, and dynamically to resolve deep problems of separation and individuation with her internalized mother from the past as well as with her real mother in the present.

---

[*] Originally published in <u>Disorders of the Self: New Therapeutic Horizons</u>, J.F. Masterson & R. Klein, eds., Brunner/ Mazel, 1995, pp. 205-226.

But just as Diana seemed ready to end a successful process of therapy, a new level of conflict emerged, as though the character work—the resolution of the false self defense—had strengthened the patient's real self to face some previously hidden part. It appeared that the borderline character structure not only had protected her in childhood from the abandonment depression, but it overlaid a dissociative response to an early traumatic experience. Once the character defense had been essentially resolved, her real self became strong enough to face and reclaim the part of the self encapsulated in the dissociated response to the trauma, and to manage the pain of accepting that "lost" part.

This led to a period of intensive work focused on recovery of this traumatic material (two to three sessions a week for seven months). The final working-through stage required management of residual character work; the experiencing of early, buried trauma; and the integration of both into a reconstruction of her life story and sense of self that was perceptually convincing and emotionally transformative. After two additional years of this working through, she was aware that her sense of self was healing, that she believed in herself and her reality.

Diana entered psychotherapy at the age of 29. At 34 years of age, she began the uncovering of the early traumatic experience, and successfully terminated treatment at the age of 38.

5.2. Issues raised by departures from classic dynamic technique

The shifts in technique required by this case raise questions regarding the role of the therapist and therapeutic neutrality, and relate to the skills, judgment, and flexibility useful in meeting the appropriate needs of the patient at the right time.

For the initial character work, the therapist had to be active, confronting the transferential acting-out distortions of the patient from a position of therapeutic neutrality. In the working-through phase, as the patient took on more responsibility for feeling and insight, the therapist became less active, limiting interventions mainly to interpretations intended to raise transference distortions to conscious awareness.

In the working through, it is the neutral, nondirective attitude of the therapist that provides the even ground that, by contrast, accentuates the patient's transferential reactions. However, in therapy with disorders of the self, it is usual to revert to active, ego-oriented interventions at times (especially as the abandonment depression emerges) to help the patient resolve regressions to old, maladaptive defenses. It is the building of an inner, dynamic structure that allows the patient to manage this technical shift in a constructive way. As Masterson (1976) has described:

> The developing alliance between the therapist's healthy ego and the patient's reality ego brings into existence, through introjection, a new object relations unit: the therapist as a positive (libidinal) object relations who approves of separation-individuation + a self representation as a capable, developing person + a "good" feeling (affect) which ensues from the exercise of constructive coping and mastery rather than regressive behavior. (p. 64)

I suspect that this strengthening of the ego and the therapeutic alliance, together with the internalization of maturing object relations, is also a critical condition for the introduction of hypnotic technique in work with dissociated events. When an isolated instance of posttraumatic stress disorder occurs in an adult with a relatively mature psyche, good basic ego strength and object-related intactness may provide a sufficient foundation for hypnotic work; in fact, the issue of transference may be a minimal one. But when the "forgotten" trauma has occurred in the developmental years, issues of arrested development need to be dealt with first, to provide the self with the capacity to "remember" that which once had to be "forgotten" so that the impaired self could survive. Perhaps still more important, issues of transference and countertransference have to be sufficiently understood and resolved so that hypnotic techniques do not contribute to anti-therapeutic fantasies.

In a case that has unfolded therapeutically as the patient's real self has grown stronger, the need for varied techniques may be called for-in response to the unfolding of the real self, and to facilitate it.

Ideally, it seems, work with forgotten trauma, or posttraumatic stress disorder, should be approached only with patients who have reached a high level of interpersonal differentiation and a sense of the real self. Unfortunately, we are too often faced with the patient whose traumatic reactions exceed his or her capacity to contain them effectively.

It might be helpful to draw a comparison between the use of medication and the use of hypnosis. The use of hypnosis as an anesthetic is a relatively accepted medical procedure, especially in the practice of dentistry and in the modification of chronic pain. Hypnotic techniques are used in these instances much as medication is used. Indeed, they are sometimes understood as a way of stimulating the brain's own self-medicating skills (for example, the production of endorphins).

The introduction of hypnotic techniques into the process of dynamic psychotherapy also raises questions reminiscent of those evoked by the administration of medicine.

The use of hypnosis as an anesthetizing containing technique is also finding acceptance in the mental health field especially in work with phobias and other anxiety states. In addition, ego-building hypnotic techniques that support self-confidence are coming into use, along with hypnotic techniques that reinforce dissociative barriers.

The use of hypnosis to anesthetize, desensitize, and contain may not have reached the level of acceptance achieved by medication, but it is relatively uncontroversial as compared with use of hypnosis as an opening-up technique, especially in conjunction with dynamic psychotherapy.

As an exploratory, experiential technique, hypnosis is being refined, scrutinized, and questioned. The case presented here is an anecdotal example of the benefit that hypnotic work can bring to a patient who has dissociated an early traumatic experience. The case also raises questions for the thoughtful clinician about the nature of memory (which to some extent is always a reconstructed, narrative phenomenon).

The presentation describes a persevering woman who was able to work selectively with hypnosis to unblock the emergence of her real self. The foundation of her endeavor was the character work and working through she pursued rigorously with the Masterson Approach. With this foundation, she believed she had the strength to hold and integrate the impact of the abuse memories she perceived to be gradually surfacing.

I do not think that hypnosis is a shortcut to revealing a disarmed impaired self in any way. However, it can be a method of supporting the unfolding of the real self that has gone through a process of strengthening its containing, observing, managing, and integrating capacities.

5.3. Character Work or Ego Repair

5.3.1. Initial Consultation

Diana came to the Masterson Group because of a separation crisis. She told me she had been "in an unhealthy relationship with a married man." She said: "I had such difficulty ending it that I was frightened. I couldn't cope with things because I was so preoccupied with my feelings." She had been depressed, with persistent fears that she would go crazy. She had experienced something similar when she graduated from college—an "overwhelming feeling of not knowing what to do." She had broken off the relationship, and she was determined to know what had happened to her.

Underlying the presenting problem were deeper separation issues. She described herself as a strong-willed and independent person, and had clashed with her father when he opposed her going away to college. She argued ferociously with her mother, who was aggrieved because Diana refused to confide in her about the affair she had just ended. But she also spoke protectively of her parents. She said that her father had eventually supported her independence, and that they were just getting to know each other in an adult way when he died suddenly of a stroke when she was 19 years old and away at college. She said that her mother always had been "really good," and that she felt close to her, and depended on her for support and approval. Although Diana had been essentially on her own for the past six years, there had been occasional periods of living with her mother.

Diana is intelligent and attractive, with golden-red hair that sweeps around her face. She combines fashionable poise with a vulnerable prettiness, and directs herself with a clear, analytical mind. In talking with her, I was interested in her paradoxical combination of childlike appeal and intellectual matter-of-factness, and mentioned this to her. She replied that people often brought this to her attention. She added that, although she looked to others for moral support, she was "critical of people-I don't give them a chance." This longing for relatedness, paired with aloofness, became a consistent indicator of her central conflict over intimacy.

5.3.2. History

Diana was the third of four living siblings. There were two older sisters, who both struggled with physical and marital problems. A third sibling, a boy, died soon after birth. Diana, born next, was a favored child who took the place of the dead brother until a younger brother was born into the family when she was four years old.

The mother, an active, opinionated woman, ran the family. All the siblings looked to her for support, and used her as a confidante even as adults. The father was somewhat more emotionally available than the mother, but less influential.

Diana described her family as ideal. Her childhood memories were vague and rosy. She thought her problems had begun with adolescence, when she became headstrong and rebellious. She had expected to float through a debutante adolescence, but felt that the magic had run out when her turn had come.

Although she fought to have her own way, she clung to romantic attachments to carry her across the transition points in her life. In her work situations, she was effective, but took a second-in-command role. As a result, she frequently was hurt and frustrated by superiors who seemed less perceptive and organized than she was. She still had not found work that truly satisfied her, although her position as a private school administrator was challenging. She dedicated herself to working with children because, as she said, she was disgusted with adults who act like children.

The diagnostic impression was of a high-level borderline disorder of the self, with separation-individuation issues and a characteristic oscillation between clinging and distancing defensive positions. Unless one paid attention to this preoedipal dynamic, it would have been easy to mistake her for neurotic, thus stalemating the treatment in some falsely compliant or hostile form of acting out.

5.3.3. Observing Ego

During the first year of her therapy, Diana's observing capacity strengthened. Intellectually, she set herself to work immediately, exploring patterns in her life. She noted that she felt like a teenager, dependent on her mother, but trying to be independent. She resented the sense of obligation she connected with dependency, and wryly remarked: "My sisters have their husbands, and I have my mother."

She began to play out her character patterns in the therapeutic relationship. She wanted me to guide her, but resisted my inquiries. I noted that she seemed to want to lean on me, but then pulled away. She told me that, after our second session, she dreamed that a woman cab driver had taken her to Trump Tower. Diana had liked her until it was time to pay, when she realized that the woman planned to shoot her. This was followed by another dream of being shot in the back by a woman friend.

The dreams were associated with trusting her feelings to a special other person. She told me that she had resisted my inquiries about her love affair, because she knew she would cry and she was afraid to let it happen. She thought relationships changed once a partner showed feeling, and remembered her mother's often saying: "Don't wear your heart on your sleeve, or they'll take advantage of you."

She began to see her childhood and her family in a new way. From the outset, I had confronted the discrepancy between her idealized account of her past and her uncertainties about her present self and relationships. It seemed puzzling that such seeming security could produce such insecurity. At first, she had said that the only upsetting event of her childhood was when the dog died. Now she viewed her life "in two places-like day and night." There was the shiny surface that was presented to the neighbors, and beneath it was a dark side marked by arguments, emotional isolation, and rebellion.

She realized that she had been frightened of her mother, who had given her the impression that love is a relationship between a powerful person and a helpless, needy one. She remembered that her mother's disapproval could make her feel as if she had been shot. She recalled her dependency on approval, and how smart and quick she had become in avoiding disapproval (she learned by watching how the middle sister was scapegoated). She also had adopted an emotional detachment that provided some distance to keep her from fears of being engulfed.

As she became more observing and insightful, she expressed herself more directly with her mother and became more assertive at work. She also began to reveal her feelings in sessions. Her real self was beginning to emerge. She choked up when describing how her life had been an illusion, and how she had learned to undermine the closeness she sought.

Tenacious preoedipal issues dominated the oedipal, which often seemed close to the surface. She dreamed that she was searching for her father, who was lost "out in the dark, out in the waves." When she tried unsuccessfully to date, she had dreams of a wave sweeping the man away. The maternal element predominated, reinforced by the father's early death.

5.3.4. Anger and Therapeutic Alliance

In the second year of therapy, Diana's detachment gave way to outbursts of anger at her mother. She also manipulated the treatment frame in a way that suggested avoidance of anger at me. She increased her sessions to twice a week, but interrupted intense sequences with illnesses and vacations. She filled her sessions with accounts of chaotic and genuinely distressing events, which tended to place the emphasis on *doing* rather than on *understanding,* and also took the focus away from our relationship.

I confronted her various ways of distancing from the sessions. I also shared some of my own induced countertransference feelings. I puzzled over my contradictory impressions of her intense dedication to the therapy and the opposite sense that she might walk away any minute, or somehow was not even there at all. She responded with both consternation and interest. She felt I had criticized her commitment, and yet she knew that she only wanted to present her efficient and intellectual side to me. As she divided her family memories into night and day, so she was dividing her therapy into superficial compliance and covert resistance.

When I asked about this double therapy, she replied that she had no clear sense of herself and was afraid of being robbed of what she had left. She recalled a recurring dream, in which she was about to be married and realized it was a terrible mistake. "Are you concerned that this therapeutic relationship might be a mistake?" She answered by telling another dream: She was trying to find her way to me through a crowded, chaotic store. We then met in my waiting room, with people coming and going. At one point, she walked out on me; at another, I took someone else into my office. In the transference, fears of engulfment and abandonment alternated.

At last, she said, she had come to terms with a transferential conflict. She had been angry that I had not given her wise advice and led her to better feelings. She was beginning to understand what psychotherapy was about, and that she was using me as a guide through a process of self change—that I could not prevent her from feeling this process was sometimes painful, but I could support her through it.

After this acknowledgment of anger at unmet dependence, she became depressed. She said she felt that she had no power, that the world was hopeless, and that she was frightened all the time. She also released some of her resentment at having to act as mother to her own family and at having to fill the father's place as the problem-solving family member as well. Diana was more open and ready to reach out. She reported that her friends found her more receptive, and I felt the same way.

5.3.5. Emergence of the Real Self

Diana had protested: "There is no room in my life for me!" During this third year, she began to change. She wanted to let go, but asked: "How can I let go without a sense of self to hold onto?"

Her dreams about water continued, and she told me that she was a capable and fearless swimmer. But, she said, she was fearful of swimming at night and did not know why. As we talked about this, the metaphor "swimming in dark water" became a way of talking about her unconscious.

As she showed more concern for herself, her interest in others increased. Her interest in men also revived.

I wondered why she dated so little when she appeared to have every advantage. She acknowledged that friends had said the same thing, but that she did not see herself as others did. She had no sense of her impact on others and described having a false self, created to comply with the family need for social approval. Inside, she felt inadequate, frightened, and absent. This inhibited self pulled away from romantic contact.

Once she identified this hidden self behind the false *facade,* she was amazed to discover how all-pervasive her anxiety actually was. The "night" side of herself was diffusely, ubiquitously afraid of everything.

5.3.6. Self-activation and Emergence of Phobia

In the fourth year of therapy, she initiated a search for a new job, and she also found a lover. He was a corporate executive who had been a silent admirer of hers for a number of years. However, he had a tendency to remain distant emotionally, even when their relationship became close, and I expressed my concern that she might be repeating her relationship with one or both parents. I wondered whether she was putting herself into the same kind of situation that first brought her into therapy, perhaps as a defense against the deepening of the process. But the couple seemed genuinely devoted to each other, and they worked hard to clarify their relationship in long, soul-searching talks.

At first, she tended to react to his unavailability with alternate clinging and rageful distancing. She recognized her acting out in time, and took a realistic stand. She told him that they would have to separate until he went into therapy to address his conflicts with relationships. Although this assertive move evoked a dream of being cut down her entire body, she held to the separation until, several months later, he entered treatment.

During this year, she also made an assertive job change. She took an executive position in which she was in charge of developing a groundbreaking program.

A dynamic change took place. Her pervasive anxiety, which had emerged when she set aside her old character defenses of avoidance and denial, now became focused in a symptom. She developed a public-speaking phobia. As she explored the phobia, it seemed to symbolize a condensation of oedipal and preoedipal issues: of forbidden self-assertion and dangerous competition with the mother.

Technically, I found myself relying more on interpretation. Earlier in the treatment, my interventions (primarily confrontation and here-and-now interpretations) had been more directed toward ego strengthening. Now I found myself dealing more with the patient's unconscious.

5.3.7. Impasse

During the fifth year, Diana developed a more separate, mature relationship with her mother. She also visited her father's grave for the first time (she is the only one in the family to have done so), She seemed substantially to have resolved inner-world issues with both parents. In addition, her view of her childhood, although disillusioned, was more real and more consistent with her understanding of her adult life. She seemed to be moving steadily to a resolution of her character issues, except that the phobia persisted.

Then she began to feel that she was carrying a terrible secret. The perception did not appear like a sudden insight, but more like vestiges of a dimly remembered dream that steadily became clearer and more convincing.

She wondered if she had been sexually molested as a child, and discussed this with her sisters. The middle sister expressed a similar anxiety, but was unable to find any basis for it in memory. Diana's lover also had intuited that she might have been molested. He observed that she had a "scared and angry look" when by herself, and tended to have childlike reactions when upset: she would shiver and her teeth would chatter.

She had dreams of having to rescue children, while her family went from room to room trying to kill them.

It was clear that the resolution of Diana's character work was releasing a deeper level of conflict. But the nature of the conflict was not clear. Diana was increasingly convinced that she might be able to access some childhood trauma through hypnosis. I thought that the speaking phobia might indicate an emerging oedipal conflict or a deeper level of conflict with the mother, and pursued both possibilities, but with poor results.

Did this impasse represent an earlier abuse or an oedipal—or even preoedipal—fantasy pressing toward consciousness? Nearly five years of solid character work had opened the door of the self, only to find another door beyond.

5.3.8. Trauma Work

In the sixth year of therapy, Diana became increasingly dissatisfied with the therapeutic process—she was no longer moving ahead. Her physical symptoms also increased: swollen lymph nodes, ovarian pain, and weight losses of five pounds at a time. Her body seemed to support her verbalized request for help. She said: "I'm trying to remember what I don't remember. I feel there's something there—inside of me—and it's blocked. It makes me have thoughts about being molested-something like that."

Neither logic nor free association could move the process. She reasoned that something might have happened to her when she was four years old, her age when the brother was born and the family was relocating.

Her mother had been emotionally overwhelmed at that time, and the patient and the middle sister had been sent to stay with an aunt and uncle. But no further thoughts came, only her sister's dream that terrorists had broken in while she was sleeping at her aunt and uncle's home.

Recollection evaded her, but her painful physical and emotional states increased. She developed sinus trouble and a cystitis-like irritation. Her legs hurt, her skin hurt. "Everything feels sensitive," she said, and then began to develop nausea and intestinal pains. She was given antibiotics for her sinus infection, but could find no other medical relief (or definitive diagnosis). She would become angry with her lover, and then with me, but the anger refused to focus: She hated everything.

As the work remained static, she turned more to her spiritual life for relief, trying to find consolation in a private world of meditation. I believed that my hesitation to explore hypnotically for deeply dissociated material was countertransferential. I wondered if I might not have assumed the role of the mother who would not make the extra effort to look at her daughter's problems, while the daughter detached herself and tried to find her own means of solace. At that point, I decided to incorporate hypnotic technique into her therapy.

5.3.9. The Preparation Phase

Contemporary hypnosis, like other current approaches to the treatment of the self, is not authoritarian; the skill of the therapist is used to facilitate the emergence of the capacities of the patient. The extensively reported work of the hypnotist Dr. Milton Erickson has revolutionized modern trance work in this way. Using the Ericksonian approach, I assured Diana that I recognized her ability to hypnotize herself—that she had developed an unconscious expertise for shifting into protective states of mind-and that I would be helping her to access this ability on a conscious level.

I began by inviting her to try a simple relaxation exercise to demonstrate that the trance state could be a pleasant one. Next, I asked her to choose a calm environment, such as a beach, and to create it clearly in her mind, using all five senses. This, I explained, was to show how resourceful her mind could be in constructing sheltering places to return to whenever she wished. After that, I suggested she explore a deeper trance state, where she would be amazed to find that she could separate her arm from her conscious will, so that it would move by itself, even though her conscious thoughts tried to hold it steady. I assisted the induction of this state by counting down from 10 to zero. When the arm moved independently, she had confirmation of her capacity for dissociative states. Last, I proposed that she return to the beach to enjoy her feelings of relaxation and discovery before coming back to full awareness of my office. I counted from one to five to help her pace this return. (The counting, to facilitate entrance into and exit from altered states, also was to help her begin to use my voice as a reinforcement at times of heightened resistance.)

Diana came to the next session feeling "terrible" and complaining in an unfocused, repetitive way. I assumed that this was a defensive resurgence of the old character work, and confronted her: "You've just taken the initiative to approach your problem from a new angle, and now you're back to waiting for someone to make things right for you." She centered herself around the confrontation, and acknowledged that she was acting out her anxiety, rather than trying to understand it. She said: "There's always something in the back of my head all the time—something that makes me afraid of exposing myself to people." She thought for a while, and then added: "I have to focus more on what I need. Basically, I just have no self-esteem."

I suggested that we work together to create a safe place, uniquely hers, that would be a haven in her inner world. (The safe-place induction is a standard procedure for therapy with trauma survivors. It is described, along with other containing techniques, by Brown and Fromm [1986, pp. 279-281].)

She chose a hilltop for this inner haven, patterned after a place to which she had gone to meditate during a retreat that had been deeply meaningful to her. The hilltop had a view across farmlands to the sea. In the induction; she would walk thoughtfully to the hill top and sit at the feet of the great stone angel that stood there.

As she began to reinforce the inner reality of the safe place, she said emphatically: "I want to keep going." She did this despite the increasing pressure of sleep disturbance, and awaking from what sleep she was able to get feeling disoriented and wanting a target for unfocused feelings of anger. The establishment of a more containing structure, cognitively and in her inner experience, offered an increased sense of safety, and so seemed to give permission for dissociated material to draw closer to her conscious awareness.

5.3.10. Crossing the Repression Barrier

There still was no spontaneous appearance of lost events. I think that when abuse and posttraumatic stress disorder have occurred during the formative years, they not only are handled by dissociation layered over by character development, but are hidden further from reach by the institution of the repression barrier. Freud equated the idea of the repression barrier with the concept of infantile amnesia, a widely observed but not altogether understood phenomenon that marks a stage of psychic growth at which memories of the first years of life fade or are forgotten. He believed that information obscured by the repression barrier became unconscious, and only tended to return if strong psychic conflicts could not be resolved. In psychoanalytic theory, that which is repressed, or is unconscious in the psyche, is accessible by a different language than that which is consciously available. Freud developed his concept of free association to help the analyst "hear" the analysand's unconscious more distinctly: the nonlinear associations of the analysand's talk—the apparently random remarks that are joined by some common denominator-constitute the primary process language that conveys the message of the repressed.

Can Freud's way of listening to the unconscious be reversed into a way of talking to it? Much has been said about Milton Erickson's use of metaphor to access a part of the mind not reached by linear, secondary process communication. I think there is more involved here than telling a story indirectly (and more pleasurably). When Erickson (1966) strengthens the physically ill gardener by making random references to the growth of a healthy garden (pp. 510-520), he is bypassing logical talk and using associative language to address the unconscious part of the mind. It seems he is using what he called the interspersal technique (1966), or what might be described as reverse associations, as a way to talk to that part of the mind that thinks in terms of space and images, and is in profound contact with feeling.

Watzlawick (1978) has described Erickson's interspersal technique in the following way:

> This intervention is essentially a dream "in reverse": What Erickson says could just as well be reported by the patient as her dream, in which consciously unacceptable material camouflages itself into the language of images in order to bypass the censorship of the left hemisphere. Of course, the important difference here is that the dream is usually the *passive* expression of inner conflict, while Erickson's use of dream language represents an *active* intervention. (pp. 62-63)

I am learning to be concerned with reverse associations when helping a patient across the repression barrier. Before using the more logical, but still unique, language of dissociation, I try to talk to the unconscious, to request passage to the inner world.

In Diana's case, I wanted to send a message to the unconscious that crossing the boundary from the hidden to the open, from the dark to the light, could be accomplished as a natural process; that, no matter how things might seem to change, all still had a safe and natural point of reference. Here is an example of how I incorporated that message, together with her personal image of safety, the stone angel, into the safe-place induction.

> *You follow the familiar path to the hilltop. The earth is solid beneath your feet, while the trees cast a changing shadow that gives way to sunlight, back to shadow and to sunlight again. And, at the hilltop, the path opens to a comfortable area where you can brush away the pebbles and twigs, and settle yourself at the feet of the angel. A line*

can move imperceptibly as the shadow of the angel moves over the clearing, and the shadow of the mountain moves across the valley. The earth shifts like a dial of shadow and sunlight, and you know it moves as it has to; as the dial of seasons always moves as it completes itself. Just as the far-off tide rises clear on the coast, and the fishing boats float free to turn on the anchor line. You can see through the clear water, down to the bits of shell and fragments of ancient cargoes, and all the sea keeps or may bring in with the tide, or carry back to its depths. Just as you see through the depths of the clear sky, where your mind wheels with the flight of the birds that see the travel far, but always carry with them the unthought knowledge of return.

Over a period of weeks, the patient seemed to wander in a region of fragmented images. These images related to childhood, and flickered by momentarily, or seemed to form the beginning of a narrative, only to fade again. There were early images of being in her crib: lonely, and sometimes drawn into a corner, seeming to take refuge in a solitude that was more reassuring than the distracted presence of her mother. There were brief impressions of driving somewhere with the family. There were recollections of the sound of a motorcycle going by at night, of falling out of bed more than once.

At first, this response seemed random and frustrating. But there was a sense of nonlinear scanning that made me wonder if the patient's images were sorting their way toward a common theme. The lonely child, the night fears, the family trip somewhere-all might be information communicated to me in the spatial, imagistic language of the unconscious. If this were so, the patient might be making her way across the repression barrier.

In the hope that I was making some contact with my patient's unconscious, I then introduced age-regression techniques. She tended to linger in the area of ages three to four:

> "I was four when we moved. There's some underlying thing of my mother's being there and not really paying attention to me . . . . My dolls are around the table for a tea party; I was happy creating things for myself . . . ." With the intensification of feeling, Diana shifted dissociatively into the use of the third person: "I'd like to take her and put her someplace else-a place to play, a place that's happy."

There followed recollections of being by the water in the summer; picking raspberries; being outdoors much of the time, and not home; feeling a distance between her parents. An image of changing her bathing suit in the summerhouse—the intrusion of a smell she did not like-the image of a face in the window.

At this point, she became frightened: "I feel like something happened in that room, but I don't know if I'm making it up." Respecting her protective withdrawal into denial, I no longer asked her about her "own" experiences. I called on her capacity to dissociate to modify her feelings: "Tell me about the four-year-old. Is there anything else you would want me to know about her on that day in that house?" "She's scared to have anyone touch her. She's afraid. She wishes somebody would hold her."

Diana had been "permitted" across the repression barrier by the internal "censor," to be in touch with a hidden, frightened child part of her self experience and self organization. It would take more than seven months incrementally to retrieve the experiences of that early time, but the door stood open.

5.3.11. Evolution of the Traumatic Experience

As we returned to the experiences of the four-year-old, coherent pictures began to form in Diana's mind, accompanied by intense, almost intolerable emotions. She said: "I feel scared and panicky. It's hard not to cry. I want to say 'Stop! I don't want to do this any more!'"

I steadily encouraged her to describe the child and the summerhouse: the quality of the light, the wallpaper, the position of the doors and windows, and the child's perception of another's presence.

She became aware of the man at the window, and his subsequent entrance through the door. She was unable to "see" his face. Realizing that increasing anxiety was reinstating dissociation, I encouraged her to use dissociation in a way that would modify the image she sought without obliterating it. "You are seeing this as if it were a photo in an old family album. The picture is very faint. It is faded with time. But you can probably make it out." As we reviewed the family album in her mind, she found a "photo" of her uncle that matched the summerhouse and the terrified feeling that was associated with it. This identification was further validated by a sense of anger and relief at the end of the session.

Session after session, the narrative moved forward incrementally, like a film strip examined without a projector.

The four-year-old put her hand to her face. The man moved forward, his face was close to hers: 'When I saw his face, I felt dizzy. Things started to spin. I can't stand his face near my face!"

Increasingly, however, the scene at the summerhouse was interrupted by flashes of another episode-the uncle entering the bedroom where four-year-old Diana and her sister were sleeping.

In successive sessions thereafter, her mind scanned back and forth between the two episodes. When she was able to recall his hand on her vagina in the summerhouse, she remembered his pulling down her pajama pants in the bedroom. Her increased tolerance for one memory seemed to open the way for the next. And, as both episodes moved to the moment when he exposed his penis, a third episode began to unfold, in which she was going down the basement stairs in her uncle's house, and he was there.

"He starts coming down, and closes the door behind him at the top of the stairs. He's talking. He says we're going to play the game again. And it's like she knows what's going to happen. It's the day after the night he came into the bedroom. He takes her arm. Pulls her down the stairs. I think he hits her. [Diana puts her hands in front of her face, and her voice becomes higher pitched.] I feel like I'm crying. Horrible, scared, panic feeling. It's worse than before, because now I know what will happen."

Her mind scanned back and forth among the three episodes as if each evoked the other, and also as if the shifting modified the escalating intensity, as she began to tell how the uncle had raped her vaginally and anally. At first, I was confused by this scanning, thinking it might be avoidance, and then began to realize that it was an unfolding process with a nonlinear logic of its own: the uncanny signature of the unconscious.

Throughout these abreactions, Diana sat opposite me, as she did in sessions generally, but in a trance, with her eyes closed. She was self-contained, holding the work largely in her mind's eye, although she was visibly in conflict and pain. Her hand often reached up to protect her face. She reported alternating disbelief and emotional pain so intense that, at times, she could not continue. Her physical symptoms corresponded to the details of the abuse, and tended to intensify and then lift as she constructed her recollections.

She was consumed by mental preoccupation and physical reaction to the work, but continued to function normally, although she said she felt as if she had to force herself to do every small task.

The impact of the work on her perception of her life was becoming significant. She said bitterly: "The worst part is to have a mother who doesn't know or understand. I can't believe it! I don't know how she didn't know!" And then: "It's a terrible sadness to realize I never had a family. I feel sad for what my mother never was; and how we all had to live in this false world."

She recalled going home as a changed person, and her mother's never noticing the difference. "I was so afraid someone was going to say something. I think that's when it started—when I started going inside my head. Where all the distancing started. I thought everyone else had those things in their heads that they didn't talk about."

5.3.12. External Validation

As Diana began to move from the uncovering of trauma to the integrating of it into her conscious life experience, she began to tell her story, first to friends, and then to her family.

When she related what had happened to the middle sister, she received a startling but confirming response. The sister responded emotionally: "I know what happened in that bedroom. I was in the bed to the right, and you were on the floor." The sister was caught up in a flashback, and sobbed uncontrollably for 15 minutes.

5.3.13. Telling the Mother

The abreactions subsided but Diana continued to feel tense: "It's something I'm controlling. It feels like the withholding of emotion."

She hesitated about revealing her memories to her mother, concerned that it would only cause more pain and distance in the relationship. A weekend with her family brought home the futility of trying to get close; they seemed cold, and she experienced the old feelings of vulnerability and isolation. "They're such a helpless lot!"

Using energy freed by the abreactive process, and perhaps also trying to offset her own feeling of helplessness, she followed through on practical goals for herself. She applied to resume her studies for a doctorate, and bought the condominium she had longed for and could now afford.

But the momentary lift in energy subsided, and finally she made the decision to break the years of silence and talk to her mother. She was pleased and perplexed by the results. Her mother was sympathetic, distressed, even angry on her behalf. She supported Diana's revelations: "I know my child. To see you in a state like this, I know it's true."

Diana was astonished at the difference that time had made in the relationship: "It's hard separating her now from who she used to be." Who the mother "used to be" was clearer, too, now that past and present could be sorted out: "I really haven't wanted her to get that close to me as an adult.

"I felt as if she possessed me, could take over my entire being, especially if it had to do with some kind of disapproval."

The old mother still lingered, though, as her present-time mother ruefully reflected: "But you were always so happy!"

5.4. Integration of Trauma and Character Work

Cathartic abreaction retrieves memory, but, alone, does not restore the self. It would take an additional two and a half years for Diana to reconcile her abuse memories with her remaining character issues of present-day identity and relationship.

The first challenge was simply to reperceive her own history. She was angry that, unknowingly, she had had to shape her character to cope with her developmental conflicts, and this, also outside of her conscious awareness, had been complicated by childhood trauma. "It's bad enough to have a problem, but worse not even to know you have it. I feel I wasn't me my whole life."

5.4.1. Past and Present Anger

On the level of dissociation, resolving her early trauma had reclaimed the lost part of herself, but also had released the last, dammed-up reservoir of abandonment depression into her consciousness.

She struggled to understand and to integrate this outpouring of hopelessness and anger without letting it slip into behavior, but she could not resist some reinstatement of the old, inadequate, defensive self: "I have a feeling of regret about my life. I feel as if everything's too late; too late to fix it."

The stuckness persisted. Her ability to grieve and let go was blocked by her defensively anchored disbelief in her own worth. Worse still, the public-speaking phobia had returned, flooding her with waves of panic. Facing a resurgence of problems she had fought for years to overcome, she remarked half-jokingly, "I could murder you."

That reaction, I thought, indicated where the conflict remained. The bond of hostile accommodation to the internalized mother of the past (as reflected in the transference) still held her back. She tentatively agreed: "I can't imagine anyone caring a lot about me. I'm just waiting to be criticized. I just hate myself, and expect everybody to tell me how awful I am. I probably don't think I have a *right* to get angry."

She began to understand that "the mother-tie is the crux. That feeling I have that nothing will get better has no real basis any more. But I can't stand the expectation of her anger-it's subtle stuff that permeates things. So I always feel wrong. I'm doing something good and then it turns out to be bad. That's the remaining problem—my fear of being intimidated. My mother's anger blows away who I am."

She began connecting patterns differently, finding past origins for feelings that seemed attached to the present. In the here and now, her anger sometimes focused on me, but especially on a female colleague of hers who held a position of authority. She expressed her anger, noted how disproportionate it was, and tracked it back to the past: "I feel like smashing you. It's consuming. Then it wants to go out of my feelings, out of my thoughts, and into my body.

I'm trying not to get sick. Why aren't you helping me? And then I realize that this is the anger I didn't feel at my mother for leaving me with my uncle."

Diana, wishing to establish her self-belief by facing the person who had damaged it, tried to confront her mother. She hoped to reach that part of her mother that knew about the undercurrent of violence and victimization in the family, and, by doing so, to free both of them from the pressure of family secrets. But her mother, now not quite hiding from herself, but too set in her ways to change, responded: "Sometimes it's too frightening to know what's in your heart."

Diana told me: "This is the first time I've really felt for her. She's let me "feel sorry for her in a strange way."

Anger was giving way to reality, leaving a growing sense of the separateness of her mother and herself, and of grief releasing the past to the realm of memory.

5.4.2. Capacity for Self-Belief

Diana observed that she now could look in a mirror and see what she really looked like, not what she hated. She was amazed to think of the state of absolute terror in which she had routinely lived. Her public speaking phobia lifted, her relationship with her lover became downgraded into that of a deep friendship, and her career began again to climb.

The old belief system, supported by the mother's emotional unavailability and absence during a critical early crisis, was losing its hold. What would take its place?

The family had used achievement as the only autonomous way to support a sense of self, but Diana was skeptical about that. "You aren't allowed to say things are just fine. The thought of doing something less than spectacular is unacceptable.

"But I'm not buying this any more. I think I'm finally all right. I used to wait for the time when everything would be perfect. Now I know I'm going to get upset and get over it."

But what was missing? Another family reunion brought the issue into focus.

"They're all shouting 'take care of me.' Everyone *needs* so much—and they need to need because needing feels like love! That's why things have to stay messed up, why this one is complaining and that one is rescuing, and why the crisis never stops!"

This insight was self-affirming, and carried her through a stressful series of interviews for a high-level executive position, during which she was repeatedly interviewed before increasingly larger groups. She maintained her confidence until the last interview, which was to be held before the entire board of directors of the organization. She became unsure, and told me: "I'm getting advice about how to talk, move, dress—but people are just telling me who to be. It's not the answer. I need to be believed in for whom I am."

I reviewed all my reasons, based on over eight years of work together, to support why I deeply believed in her capacity to handle the interview, and why, beyond that, I felt I could believe in her as a person. I realized, as I did this, that my reality-based reinforcement of her qualities as a profession and a person was a new experience for her—that the real relationship she had built with me had helped her to reinforce an internal structure that had received little previous support.

She called me to say that an outsider had been chosen for the job and that the position never really had been available to her. However, past the disappointment, she was now in a new stage of growth, spurred on by enthusiastic responses from board members who had been impressed by her and by her own feeling of having done well and having been herself.

5.4.3. Termination

As the nine-year mark of therapy approached, Diana wound down her work with me. She continued to hear from friends and colleagues how her personality had become warmer and more open. She maintained the devotion and support of a group of close friends, including her former lover. She was well on her way to completing her doctorate, and had found that her exceptional handling of the interview had brought her to the attention of a sophisticated job market.

She was amazed to find that she was not living in daily fear: "I remember when I told you I was in an elevator and realized I didn't have to be afraid of the elevator man-not everybody has a gun!"

Another family reunion had focused her emotional separation from them: "The whole *detached* lot was there, but there was no group. Everyone is afraid or angry about what everyone else is thinking. It's bizarre. There's nothing there except serving and doing. Why don't they *see?*"

She felt there was no sense of unfinished business. However, she mused: "I'm being too intellectual about leaving! It's nine years-a long time-but this therapy saved my life. You've been my only consistent anchor point for nine years."

We reflected together over those years and the process of the therapy itself. I talked about the vulnerable self that hides behind one defensive shield after another, and how skillfully she had hidden herself.

"That touches what happened when I didn't get the job! I put myself on the line with nowhere to hide. If I didn't get the job, I'd have to see if I could believe in myself, anyway. And I could. My belief in myself is real!"

With that statement, some barrier between us dissolved, and the emotional paradox of a good therapeutic closing—combined pleasure and sadness-was also real.

5.5. Epilogue

A few months after the close of her therapy, Diana contacted me with affirming news. She had been appointed to a substantial and competitive position in a major organization. She was pleased with the results of her perseverance, and especially with the loyalty of her friends and colleagues, who had supported her and whose warmth she now felt freer to accept and return.

CHAPTER 6

DISORDER OF THE SELF, TRAUMA AND THE USE OF HYPNOSIS*

I thought I would begin by retelling an old story:

> The man's name is Oedipus, and although at first he is in flight from what he believes are his own origins, some deeper drive directs his journey to the very place where his story actually began. He does not recall how his life started, but the unconscious need to return there is as deep as his need for an identity. To fill this need, he will have to find a way to tell his whole story.

> Thebes was his birthplace, but this is not remembered by him as he sets his sandaled foot

---

*Presented at *Disorders of the Self: New Therapeutic Horizons,* a conference given in honor of the works of James Masterson, M.D., and sponsored by the South African Institute for the Study of Psychoanalytic Psychotherapy and the Masterson Institute for Psychoanalytic Psychotherapy, Pretoria, South Africa, 2008.

on the red earth of the Theban plain. Suddenly, he is met with an apparition that blocks his path. A Sphinx confronts him with her great span of golden wings, her body of a lioness, the dazzling face of a woman, and the voice of a mother lion intoning softly to her cub. In the manner of such apparitions, she asks a riddle and, as the ritual goes, his life will depend of his answer.

Here is the Sphinx's riddle:

"What is it that goes on four feet in the morning, two feet in the afternoon, and three feet in the evening?"

And Oedipus replies:

"The answer is Man—for he crawls on all fours as an infant, walks on two legs as an adult, and walks with two legs and a staff in old age."

The correct answer destroys the Sphinx, and Oedipus is free to proceed to search for his origins.

Why is the answer correct? Oedipus has understood that he will survive only if he can describe the whole passage of a human life. In the legend, the Sphinx will eat him if he does not know the right answer. In the metaphor, his spirit will be devoured by a disowned and incoherent existence. The passage through the Gates of Thebes is opened by his ability to understand that the advancing stages of life lead to a sense of identity: that there is a narrative to life that provides the progression that culminates in individual meaning.

It is a human truth that we weave an identity from narrative. Apparently, the world presents us with a more or less miscellaneous sequence of events, some unpredictable, some inevitable, a few controllable. We bring to this our pattern-making minds with a need that goes beyond the intellectual. We need to make a coherent story of it all.

You might say our sense of self comes from a series of interlocking narratives. We create a narrative for how the earth was made, and within that tell the history of our tribe or nation. Within that is the account of how our family evolved, and at the center of all stories, the personal tale of the storyteller.

The human voice weaves these narratives together. Myths, epics, fairy tales, personal reminiscences take form through the human voice. Unless there is a storyteller and an audience, there is no story. Before we see our mother's face, we hear her voice, and our crowning maturational accomplishment is to be able to tell our story meaningfully to others.

Freud thought that the full expression of the self to another brings about the healing of the soul. Freud called his new science "soul-analysis," and taught that the soul is restored by the telling of one's life story to the analyst—by an "anamnesis," or process of unforgetting of the half-remembered or unaccepted parts of our lives. We are healed when we bring to full consciousness the hidden places in our life's history, and recount them to another.

We need to believe our story is credible in order to fulfill ourselves. The psychoanalyst Erik Erikson named our culminating maturational challenge the achievement of "ego integrity" over "despair"—the need to have our lives make sense in order to make our lives whole.

Nowadays, there are fewer places where we can practice telling our story. The storyteller himself is becoming a mythical figure, and families rarely get together to hear their elders reminisce. The voice of the bedtime story is giving way to mechanical devices that enchant but do not engage the child and the elder in a place of interpersonal exploration. John Bowlby and the attachment theorists are concerned, as are those in interpersonal schools of therapy, as to how we can construct a healthy basis for the continuity of the self. And one wonders especially nowadays, when the human voice, with its interchange of questions and answers, is replaced by passive observation and a television screen.

Psychotherapy has become one of the few places where there is time and encouragement for one to build a coherent life narrative in the presence of a fully receptive listener.

Patients come to therapists with a need, often unspoken, to integrate the fragmented narrative of their lives. It could be said they come to use words to restore a broken soul.

The patient with a personality disorder cannot tell a consistent, meaningful story of his or her life, since words and recollections are lost in the fear of painful emotion, and are blocked by such primitive resistances as denial, acting out, or dissociation.

Patients who suffer from psychic trauma, even more, "have had the evolution of their lives checked" (as Pierre Janet once said). These patients come to us with blocked or intrusive memories, and need to find a containing narrative for them.

As Wilfred Bion observed, the therapist waits with questions, like the Sphinx. The process proceeds with a deep sense of peril, for every silence is threatening until the patient is able to face feeling, synthesize the answer, and claim his integrated definition of himself.

———∿∿~⊙∘⊀⊙⊙⊀∘⊙∿∿———

I would like to offer a case illustration to show the importance of the therapy patient's developing a meaningful life narrative. In this case, the presenting problem was a traumatic event, and the work was complicated by cultural difference and characterological resistance. The therapy required the use of psychodynamic and cognitive interventions, as well as some hypnotherapy and, over all, the building of a hard-won and trusting relationship.

Mr. K, an elderly man, had been born in East Bengal while it was still a part of India. During the partition of India and Pakistan, he and his family had fled to Hindu West Bengal, and he grew up in Calcutta, where his father, once a well-to-do merchant, struggled to rebuild his business. Later, after the death of his father, Mr. K and his wife emigrated to the United States, where they raised a family. In his late sixties, Mr. K left the care of the business to his eldest son, and spent his time tutoring English and devoting himself to prayer.

Mr. K lived in an Indian community in a suburban area. Especially since his retirement, he had taken to wearing traditional Bengali dress: kurta and dhoti, or draped trousers with a long overshirt made of homespun material. It was this attire that, one night, made him the target of post 9/11 paranoia. (It was 2001—the time of the terrorist plane attack on the World Trade Center in New York.) A group of wandering teenagers, high and looking for trouble, saw Mr. K in his Indian dress, and ignorantly decided he was a Moslem terrorist. They taunted him, then beat him, until the timely arrival of a patrol car scattered them. Mr. K was not critically injured—the appearance of the police had saved him—but he was briefly hospitalized for his injuries, and was deeply shaken emotionally.

In the ensuing months, he lost sleep or awoke screaming that he was being attacked. He constantly replayed the scene of the assault in his thoughts, was alarmed at any sudden noise, and consistently showed these symptoms of Posttraumatic Stress Disorder. His priest encouraged him to pray, yet this only helped while he was praying. His doctor prescribed an SSRI and a minor tranquillizer, but these provided minimal relief. His family was distraught and his wife was growing hysterical. Finally, and much against Mr. K's inclination, the family (supported by the priest and the doctor) persuaded him to seek help through psychotherapy.

In my office, Mr. K presented himself as a thin, elderly Hindu gentleman—he was courteous, high-strung, of medium-brown complexion, and wearing his native Bengali dress.

He told me with polite composure that he had come in order to please his family, and hoped I would not take long to do whatever I had to do.

I explained that it was my main responsibility to be an attentive listener, and that he would help himself by telling me about himself, and especially about the assault.

He balked. "You are thinking I am a foolish old man who has gone out of his head." "I think you are an innocent citizen who has been wronged, and what happened has caused you too much pain to forget."

He seemed to relax a little, and then asked me for my credentials. "You are not a medical doctor?"

No, I responded, it was not necessary to be a medical doctor to be a trained psychotherapist. And, I added, it was a good thing for him to feel free to ask any other questions he had about psychotherapy, or myself as a psychotherapist.

He expressed doubts that I could be interested in hearing his "wild tale," or understand his feelings of humiliation.

I realized we would have to deal with cultural issues as well as his personal resistances before he could feel comfortable participating in the work.

So I said: "It is probably difficult for you to talk to a woman, especially one who is not Indian. Possibly you had hoped I would be a wise old man with a long beard like Tagore."

He laughed in surprise, and was pleased to hear my familiarity with the Bengali philosopher-poet.

"How do you know of Tagore?"

I told him of my stay in India, and especially my visit to Tagore's sanctuary, Shantiniketan. Soon we were talking about India, where I had stayed with Indian friends, eaten Indian food, and worn Indian dress.

"So you are familiar with my attire?"

Yes, I replied, and asked him if the homespun material he wore was "khadi," the material spun by Gandhi. He assented, again pleased to find that his culture was not strange to me. I added that it was a great irony that he should have been attacked for wearing attire that represented non-violence.

My observation touched his emotions, and he began to speak bitterly of the assault—not only because of its brutality, but for the injustice of attacking him as a Moslim.

I carefully remarked that this was probably especially painful because of the communal strife between Hindus and Moslems.

Candace Orcutt, PhD

He said: "Moslems drove me from my home as a child."
I remained gravely sympathetic, saying nothing, but sharing
his silence and deep feeling.

As we continued to talk, Mr. K showed indications of a
narcissistic personality disorder—not just feeling expected
vulnerability from the assault, but revealing narcissistic
vulnerability when it came to finding his experience and
symptoms under scrutiny by another. He defended himself
from this feeling of vulnerability by questioning the entire
process of therapy and my capacity as a therapist.

I continued to meet his narcissistic avoidance with
interventions that addressed his underlying sense of
vulnerability. The essential formula for such interventions
is (1) recognition of psychic pain, (2) identifying how the
patient is defending against the pain and, (3) pointing out
that the defense is intended to protect the self.

For instance, I said to him: "It is so painful to have
gone through your experience, and so uncomfortable to tell
it to a woman, that you avoid speaking of your suffering
by minimizing it, or questioning whether it is worthwhile
telling it to me."

He then said: "How can speaking with you relieve my
sleeplessness, my nightmares?"

I replied: "Even though talking is known to help such
symptoms, still, talking about them causes you pain. So you
hope to avoid the pain by avoiding the talking."

He said: "And where do you find the wisdom to help
me when even my priest cannot?" I responded: "Your priest
has spiritual wisdom far beyond mine. What I offer you
is something else—training in a scientific process that is
an established approach to eventually ease your suffering."
And I added a cognitive intervention to prepare the way
for trauma work, which benefits from a more direct,

intellectual approach: "Perhaps you think I claim some ability that is superior to your own ability to overcome your suffering yourself. But actually, it will be your own courage to face your pain and tell your story that will renew your perspective and confidence. I am only the listener who is trained to encourage you to speak despite your pain."

As time went on, I observed that Mr. K was finding it easier to talk with me. In fact, as the cultural and characterological barriers to our relationship weakened, he became quite talkative. With defenses lightened, Mr. K showed a gregarious, inquiring side to his personality that deepened our relationship and promoted the work.

He also showed a sense of humor, and his criticism of me became a more gentle teasing. He would say: "How is my little sister today? Is she ready to hear more wise thoughts from her older brother?"

As the introductory phase of the treatment deepened, Mr. K began to accept me as sympathetic, but still resisted the idea of therapy, and of myself as therapist.

He protested: "Why should I repeat this unpleasantness to you? It is humiliating." "Because a shameful thing was done to you, you believe you should be ashamed." (This was a cognitive intervention aimed at reframing his sense of humiliation.)

"Still, why should I speak of such unpleasantness?" (He remained in defense, so I returned to addressing his narcissistic vulnerability.)

I replied: "It causes you such pain to speak of this, that you protect yourself by choosing to be silent."

This time he did not avoid the issue: "It is true. It pains me to talk about this, even though it goes through my head over and over again."

Since he was no longer in defense, I returned to a more cognitive explanation: "It is often helpful in psychotherapy to tell what happened to you to a professional who will listen to what you have experienced."

"How is this of any help?"

"We find that telling your experience, and allowing yourself to express the feelings you have, helps to relieve the symptoms that are disturbing you."

As he became more familiar with talking with me, and more open, I continued to acknowledge him on three levels: First, I respected his culture; Second, I acknowledged his sense of vulnerability and even displeasure in having to face his pain with me (dealing with the personality defenses); and Third, I increasingly offered common-sense, cognitive responses to his reactions to the assault whenever he was willing to discuss it (beginning to deal with the trauma).

I believe if I had not been willing to approach Mr. K on these levels, and basically in this order, our sessions would have stopped.

Here, I would like to stress the importance of honoring these levels, which essentially means addressing strata of resistance in the treatment.

For psychotherapy is, in large part, the removing of obstacles that impede the patient's integration of a coherent life history. In order to create such a narrative for himself, Mr. K had to overcome this progression of resistances.

The first, as I have said, is the level of cultural bias. It was very difficult for Mr. K to perceive a white, female social worker as someone he could relate to as a helpful authority. It was necessary to verbalize this problem immediately, and for me to demonstrate that I respected his culture, and show that I respected him, as well—that I made no claim to superiority (only access to a skill), and regarded him as a wise elder with the capacity to find his way to his own solutions. Initially, he complained: "This is like going to a younger sister for advice." Instead of arguing, and although it was difficult to put my own pride aside, I was able to say: "I do not presume to advise you, but if your younger sister can hear her older brother express his grief to her despite his pain, then I hope I am like her." In time, he was able to remark: "You remind me of my younger sister, who is a good listener to my thoughts."

The next barrier to the treatment was the resistance created by Mr. K's narcissistic personality disorder. It was important for his therapy that he not perceive treatment as an additional form of humiliation. Talking about the attack was mortifying for him to discuss with anyone, for he was repelled by his sense of helplessness. Defining my own role was important, for, on the one hand, I could be seen as a naive younger sister, but on the other, I could be perceived as alien—uncomfortably reminiscent of some condescending colonial authority. It was crucial to see me as an enabler—someone dedicated to helping him recognize and implement his own powers of self-healing. As Dr. Masterson has defined it: I was "a servant of a process" who could guide him past his pain to find his own strength. I could explain this to a point, but had to demonstrate it convincingly by remaining neutral and appropriate in my interventions.

I had to overcome the countertransferential pull to go on the defensive and protest or lecture, for to do so would be to become the condescending, authoritarian figure he disliked.

So, when he said: "I am just a poor, brown Indian. Why should you be bothered with my problems?"

I could have replied: "Why can't you trust me?" Or "You must learn not to put yourself down." Or (still worse) "But some of my best friends are Indian!"

Instead, I fortunately answered: "This is especially hard for you, since I remind you of others who have mistreated you. I think you humble yourself before I can do it."

Apparently, this mirroring interpretation of narcissistic vulnerability was therapeutic (you never know, as Dr. Masterson says, until you hear the patient's response), for he said: "You surprise me. You talk about my thoughts as if you know me well."

These first two levels of resistance—of culture and personality type—can be difficult to meet with, as the work involves the establishment of trust and alliance. In the case of this patient, I was constantly struggling with countertransference reactions, as these forms of resistance reinforced each other to evoke feelings of inadequacy and faint guilt in me.

The third level of resistance is the block set up by the trauma itself. The patient may be eager to be rid of such trauma symptoms as nightmares, flashbacks, and a sense of helplessness, but facing the feelings associated with the trauma is itself painful. Integrating the experience into the personal narrative is hard work. In fact, if trauma work is not carefully done, and not approached on the base of a secure alliance, the patient may shut down or even become retraumatized.

A good enough atmosphere of safety is crucial in working with traumatized patients. By definition, trauma is caused when a person's defensive system is overwhelmed, and therefore it is essential to strengthen and build the patient's damaged or insufficient capacity to cope. This is why a careful assessment of personality, of character strength, must come first. Work with disorders of the personality—character work—must precede trauma work (and interweave with it when necessary) in order to prepare the patient to integrate the trauma without once more being overwhelmed. Character work, or work with a patient's defensive system, is a way of talking together that creates, over time, a sense of understanding and basic trust that allows for the exploration of the traumatic feelings that have threatened the stability of the self.

Under ideal circumstances, the patient will begin to discuss traumatic material when the therapeutic setting feels safe enough to do so. That is: when the patient feels sure enough of the relationship with the therapist to deal with material that is frightening and even humiliating.

What is work with trauma? Basically, it is enabling the patient to talk about the traumatic experience, describe it in detail, and live it emotionally. Eventually, traumatic experiences become memories that are part of the person's life experience—part of the personal narrative that contains and integrates the patient's overall life history.

Trauma work is heavily cognitive. So it is important to share with the patient exactly what I have just described to you. Trauma work, maybe more so than character work, is a consciously shared venture. The therapist invites the patient to explore the source of symptoms, acknowledges that it is difficult and painful, and enlists the patient's cooperation in reviewing the traumatic event or events.

This phase of the work is especially challenging, for the therapist usually is accustomed to being to some degree a "blank screen"—an anonymous listener who does not explain or directly guide the therapeutic process.

Working with trauma, and especially using hypnotic interventions, raises questions about therapeutic neutrality.

It is somewhat similar to being both the talking therapist and the person providing medication. If one plays a dual role, it should be treated as a parameter to the treatment—that is, a matter that needs to be discussed in its own right.

In any event, it is axiomatic for trauma work that what the therapist is doing should be clear to the patient, with no mystery about it. Trauma itself is a mystery to the patient: an obliterating happening that wipes away reason and leaves the self at the mercy of overwhelming forces. Therapy should bring understanding and a sense of control, or it will contribute to the patient's feeling of helplessness.

In trauma work, we help the patient to recount a painful, terrifying, and disorganizing experience. And again, it is useful to acknowledge exactly that in the therapy. The therapist will repeatedly say: "Recalling what happened to you stirs up frightening, almost intolerable feelings. So let me know what pace is right for you—when you want to slow down, or even take a break for awhile. Then let me know when you feel safe enough to continue."

At points where the patient chooses to hesitate, reassure the patient that the patient knows instinctively when to pause and consolidate the work. At such a point, instead of continuing to encourage description of the traumatic experience, help the patient to transform resistance into a sense of control.

Usually, the resistance has to do with intense feelings. The patient needs to discuss these. But sometimes the patient will go into a character defense, and the therapist must temporarily shift gears.

Mr. K, when describing the assault, sometimes stopped and said:

"This upsets me very much. I don't want to talk about it."

To this direct statement, I could make a cognitive reply: "People often feel this way when talking about what happened. Give yourself time to adjust to the feeling, and let's try to understand that better before you continue."

But sometimes he halted because of a more characterological resistance, and I would address his prickly sense of narcissistic vulnerability rather than hesitation caused by the sensations aroused by the trauma itself.

He would say: "I am a foolish old man to talk about such nonsense."

Then I would mirror and interpret his defensive position by saying: "It is uncomfortable for you to discuss these matters, so you dismiss them by calling them the folly of age."

I would not, in either case, return to the telling of the trauma until he was clearly ready to do so.

To return to the process of Mr. K's sessions . . . . Mr. K, in time, began to tell me about the pleasant memories he had of his childhood and of his family. He had relatives scattered throughout India, Canada, and the United States, and they visited each other with some frequency. He seemed to be becoming satisfied that I was a sympathetic listener for whom he began to feel some warmth. He knew I respected his culture, his person, and his pain.

Then one day he spoke to me openly, but in an unaccustomed shy manner.

"This talking is good for me. I feel you understand me. I like to hear your voice when you tell me not to be ashamed, and I like it when we share our tales of India."

And then: "My son tells me that you might be able to offer me some meditation that I might recall at times when I am in distress. Is that possible?"

I could not have been more receptive to the idea, and silently thanked Mr. K's perceptive son for providing me with a smooth introduction to a frequently-used hypnotic process often referred to as a Safe Place process. It is an exercise especially helpful in work with trauma survivors. It consists of constructing, together with the patient, a profoundly experienced peaceful place in the mind. It can be used as an anchor point at any time the patient needs to counteract a sense of distress with a sense of tranquility. Although the Safe Place is created in the therapy office, the patient can recreate it whenever he or she wants to reinforce or restore a sense of calm. Referring to the process as a meditation, or relaxation exercise, is accurate enough, as these are all names for a trance state that can be effective and even quite deep, and should always be induced with care and respect.

In preparation for the session, I asked Mr. K what he would consider to be a peaceful place.

"The ocean. Can you offer me a meditation about the ocean?"

Since Mr. K prayed daily, it was easy enough to encourage him to compose himself receptively for this intervention.

In the beginning, I simply introduced him to the process, assuring him that I was only a guide for his own meditative ability, and that my voice would always remain with him as a path back to the office. That he could choose to continue or stop while the session progressed.

We began with his constructing his own beach through all five senses—the rhythmic sound of the waves, the scent and taste of salt on the tongue, the endless expanse of shifting water, the cool breeze, and the heat of the Indian sun. For a few sessions he was content with deepening this meditation, recreated it during private moments at home, and claimed it brought him a sense of calm when assailed by frightening thoughts.

One day I asked Mr. K for permission to extend the Safe Place meditation to a story that might deepen his sense of calm, and he was interested in this experiment. I had worked outside the sessions to construct a hypnotic tale that would suggest that experiences of conflict, even danger, could be refrained in a supportive, even heroic narrative that would be compatible with Mr. K's world. It was important, in forming this story, to use elements that would be familiar and reassuring to Mr. K, but only to suggest a meaning and avoid the didactic. In the manner of the hypnotherapist, Milton Erickson, the story would be so structured that only the narrative would engage the left brain, while implied meaning would be directed to the intuitive right brain of the patient. In this way, the "message" would be received primarily on the unconscious level, which is more open to suggestion and affective connection.

In the story, which I elaborated at some length, I told of Mahatma Gandhi's long march to the ocean to gather salt in defiance of the British Salt Tax. I described the hardships of the long, over two hundred miles walk to the shore at Dandi, and how the marchers, at first just a few, were joined by hundreds of others, passively resisting any opposition, and finding increasing strength in their numbers and determination to reach the sea. Then, on the shore, Gandhi began to dry sea water in the sun to retrieve particles of ocean salt. At first there were only a few grains, but as the people worked together, they drew. handfuls of white crystals from the shoreline. Despite all hardship and opposition, Gandhi had peacefully defied the oppressor, and the sea had offered up its treasure to him.

Mr. K was pleased and calm. Indirectly I had suggested to him an identification with his hero—passively overcoming hardship and fear. I hoped this would help to act as a counterweight to his traumatic experience, helping to turn a sense of defeat and humiliation into a sense of perseverance and courage.

Not only did Mr. K find solace in the "story," but a strange turn of events occurred.

Shortly after the session, he told me that the meditation had had an unexpectedly healing effect on him.

Gandhi's march, he told me, had brought back the memory of his family's long flight from East to West Bengal. The journey was dangerous, and at one point some of the travelers had been attacked by bystanders—his father had been beaten to the ground. But others in the group came to their rescue, and helped them to continue.

"I felt great shame for my father," said Mr. K. "And then, when I myself was recently beaten, I felt I had been shamed like him. But as I was meditating the other day, I realized my father had nothing to be ashamed of. He took a beating, yes, but he brought us all to safety despite it. I was beaten for stating my beliefs in the way I dressed. I still make my statement and have nothing to be ashamed of."

Through this memory and the insight it brought, Mr. K transformed himself from victim to idealistic survivor. The sense of helplessness that had immobilized and overcome him began to fade, along with a sense of shame that reached far back into his childhood. His father had persisted, like those who had marched with Gandhi, and he was like his father.

His symptoms modified. Some, like the nightmares, happened less often, and he was less subject to intrusive thoughts. He could now speak of the traumatic event to others, and did not avoid it. His startle response was still pronounced, but was less easily invoked. The family was relieved and happy to see him take interest in life around him once more.

This turning-point did not take effect all at once. Mr. K spent many sessions recounting the presenting trauma. But he also dwelt on the flight to West Bengal—it actually had been an early trauma that set the stage for the later one. As he traced the years of travel and survival, his positive feelings grew for both his father and himself. "We came to the ocean," he concluded, "and we gathered the salt of life."

Here I would like to add some thoughts about trauma, dissociation, and hypnosis.

The use of hypnotic interventions, like the prescribing of psychotropic medication, is a skill, even an art, that requires training and practice. Hypnosis is a way of accessing that part of the mind that is not conscious. Therefore, hypnosis is a way of speaking to the unconscious mind in order to retrieve what has been forgotten, or in the case of trauma, dissociated. Or—as is my focus today, it can be used to shore up and even build ego strength.

Let us take a look at the relationship between trauma and dissociation. Traumatic dissociation occurs when a person directly experiences or observes an event that is perceived as so terrible that the person's usual capacity to cope with what is happening is overwhelmed. Dissociation then occurs, which is a protective mechanism that stops the mind from allowing full conscious recognition of the traumatic happening. If dissociation did not occur, the person would suffer some degree of mental collapse. Dissociation is like a circuit-breaker that prevents the mind from short-circuiting in the face of traumatic overload.

We sometimes mistakenly speak of dissociative "forgetting." It is more likely that dissociation prevents a perception from becoming fully formed. The process of so-called "remembering" traumatic events is actually the completion of an arrested process of perceiving. It could be said that the resolution of dissociation does not recover a memory—instead, it completes a memory by permitting the stored dissociated elements of the memory to integrate into conscious awareness.

It is easy to see dissociation at work when the patient is unable to recall traumatic events. It is more complex to understand when the patient has intrusive experiences, or flashbacks, of the trauma. Although such phenomena are vivid and often persistent, they remain detached from the ordinary flow of consciousness. They are fragmentary and do not integrate into the patient's life narrative (if they could do so, they would become true memories and lose their intensity over time). Flashbacks and other intrusive phenomena are unassimilated replays of traumatic events that remain dissociated from the present and from each other. They will remain so until the patient has the ego strength to fully acknowledge what happened, and weave the conscious experience of it into the overall experiencing of a life's history.

How do words, used hypnotically or otherwise, resolve the dissociative defense and facilitate the integration of traumatic experience? Essentially, words must be used to resolve resistances by reinforcing and building more effective adaptive defenses. To go back to the circuit-breaker analogy, we must aid the patient to overcome the fear of restoring the circuit by helping him to strengthen the wiring that will enable the circuit to operate safely without overloading. The therapist should not push through defenses or overload the patient's consciousness by forcing the experiencing of traumatic material. To do so would be similar to disabling the breaker before the short circuit had been compensated for.

Resolving resistances and strengthening constructive defenses: how does that work in the therapy? In the case of Mr. K, the patient had mobilized strong resistances based on culture, personality, and a need for emotional security in order to avoid the pain of humiliation, shame, and emotional disorganization. The establishment of the therapeutic alliance formed the essential foundation for the work. Addressing and easing Mr. K's suspicions that therapy might somehow prove degrading was challenging, and took up many sessions, but it formed the basis of trust necessary to approach the presenting problem. Problems of culture and character were recurring issues of resistance, and had to be responded to appropriately whenever they returned. But with the therapeutic alliance in place, there was space to begin the cognitive and hypnotic work that addressed the trauma.

Today, I would like to describe a hypnotic process that is particularly useful in treating trauma survivors, and which I touched upon in telling of the work with Mr. K. The purpose of this process is to create a Safe Place in the mind. The process can be used to promote a feeling of security in the patient, but it should also be introduced as a tool that the patient can use to anchor and re-anchor a sense of calm whenever that is needed—outside sessions as well as during them. Incidentally, some trauma survivors will say that no safe place exists anywhere. With these patients, the therapist can suggest that the patient can "Begin to create a safe place."

The Safe Place can be introduced as a hypnotic exercise, or as a meditation, or as a relaxation exercise—whatever term is most comfortable for the patient. It requires no formal hypnotic induction, although the patient may be encouraged to take a comfortable position and draw a deep breath or two. Closing the eyes is helpful, but not altogether necessary.

The Safe Place should be "created" with maximum collaboration with the patient. At no point should the process feel like an authoritarian imposition. I try to follow the principles of hypnosis put forward by Milton Erickson. The process should proceed with the patient feeling in control: choice of place should be the patient's; the patient should be assured that it is his or her unconscious that is in charge and is wise; and the patient's style of thinking should be kept in mind (is the patient more responsive to visual or auditory descriptions, etc.). And throughout, the therapist assumes the tone of a storyteller, weaving pertinent metaphors into a narrative that engages the listener.

Mr. K chose an ocean beach to be his Safe Place. We discussed it for awhile, establishing the temperature, time of day, and other details he found congenial. I was interested in working with him to create a beach that would be a concept he could visit at any time to find a sense of security. I was also interested in encouraging a sense of safety that would support his approach to traumatic material. For the therapeutic goal of this exercise is to promote the feeling that there is space in the mind to counterbalance threatening things. Throughout, the therapist is only a voice that forms a safety-line between the trance state and everyday reality.

Here is an abbreviated example of a Safe Place process. Note that the exercise only progresses with the patient's permission, that an anchor to present time is emphasized, all senses are called into operation, and the therapist speaks in a calm tone of voice:

"With your permission, I invite you to the beach you have been telling me about. Come with me now to enjoy the peacefulness you enjoy there. As you roam along the shore, my voice will go with you. My voice will always be there to invite you to enjoy your beach, or to offer you a pathway back to the here and now in my office.

"Let me invite you to walk along the shore. The sense of this beach is so calm, you know you can always come here to find a place of safety in your mind. Look out to the ocean—how peaceful it is—blue and grey as the waves rise and fall. And beyond the ocean, that barely visible line where the sea joins the grey-blue sky. Perhaps you only know there is a horizon because of the one white sail that rides along it.

"The ocean brings a fresh morning breeze to your skin. You scent the salt air and taste it on your tongue. At your feet, the water washes in, translucent at the tide-line, Under the water's edge you see the shapes and forms of shells and bright pebbles that remind you of other things. Sometimes you are reminded of their sharp edges, but all is being smoothed, being washed away by the tide. And you know your unconscious is wise and will bring you only things that are comforting for you to know.

"Perhaps you have wandered along the tide-line enough for now. Let me invite you back to present time in this room. Follow my voice and let yourself be in this room, bringing with you a deep sense of calm and thoughts of things that will surprise and delight you."

Of course, this is only a brief version of a process that can be elaborated for as long and deeply as it is useful. Watch your patient, the regularity of the patient's breathing, and note any restlessness that might indicate that you should bring the exercise gently to a close.

Again, the Safe Place process is only introduced with the patient's permission, and with the understanding that its purpose is to provide an exercise that will bring calm, and that the patient can use at any time to promote a sense of safety. The patient should be encouraged to enjoy the exercise at home, and the therapist may even give the patient a tape of the exercise to take away from the office. It also should be kept in mind that trauma survivors are often in an altered state and are particularly open to suggestion. So it is wise to be certain that your patient is not in an altered state at the end of the session. Ask how your patient feels, and suggest the patient focus on the far, middle, and near distance before ending the hour. Start talking about everyday things, and observe whether your patient is with you.

Exercises such as the Safe Place process, and any other meditative exercise aimed at calm and relaxation, can be used by someone with an average training in hypnosis. However, any hypnotic procedure directed toward traumatic material, and especially the uncovering of traumatic material, should only be attempted after the therapist has received extensive training and has had experience under qualified supervision.

Hypnosis should always be used with training and caution, but especially in work with trauma patients. As I have mentioned, trauma patients are never far from an altered state, and altered states may bring forth more than either therapist or patient bargained for. The expression of trauma may elicit further levels of trauma that have been hidden by defense.

An example of this is Mr. K's bringing forth traumatic recall of his father's being beaten. But bigger surprises than this may wait in the unconscious once a process of uncovering has begun.

Hypnosis, as a tool for working with traumatic material itself, may be used to therapeutically guide the patient through abreaction (that is, a living-through of traumatic events). Or the patient may be regressed hypnotically to reveal hidden traumatic happenings in childhood. These are specialized uses of trance that are beyond the scope of this presentation. Today I have chosen to describe that use of trance that reassures, reinforces, and even builds the patient's capacity for containing and integrating traumatic experience.

Finally, a reflection on the use of hypnosis for ego-building . . . .

The human narrative, according to Erik Erikson, begins in the foundation of basic trust. Although it must be synthesized with the therapeutic alliance, the use of hypnosis can facilitate the growth of this stage of psychic development. It would seem that we can use hypnosis to encourage dormant feelings that were hampered in their development because of a lack of secure personal attachment. Milton Erickson, the master hypnotist, demonstrated that this was possible with his "February Man" process. Erickson used his hypnotic skills to foster a sense of interpersonal caring in a young woman whose adulthood was compromised by a traumatic childhood. Erickson induced the sense of a kindly uncle who visited her on February every year her childhood, thus providing her with the feeling continuity of interpersonal concern and trust.

This longing to interrelate and trust, I believe, is unquenchable, even when hidden. It forms the basis for therapeutic work, even as it forms the opening of our life story. We probably cannot survive without it.

By way of a final illustration, I would like to describe a segment of my work with Elizabeth, a patient diagnosed with Multiple Personality Disorder, or Dissociative Identity Disorder. She came to therapy with a traumatic history of severe abuse, neglect, and very little foundation for basic trust.

Elizabeth, the primary, or host personality, typically suffered from personality disorder—she was what Dr. Masterson would call a closet narcissist, or someone whose sense of vulnerability hampers their interpersonal interaction. Initially, Elizabeth was mostly mute, and could only be encouraged to speak by such interventions as: "It is so painful for you to open your thoughts to another, that you protect yourself with silence." Such interventions eventually brought forth an alternate child personality, Beth, who reached out for the very connection Elizabeth feared: basic trust. Beth wanted me to tell her a story.

So, as I worked with the personality disorder of the primary personality, I tried to devise a way to turn Beth's love of stories into a connection that would somehow reach this dissociated part of the self that had preserved the capacity for relatedness. I decided to tell Beth a story that would include her, and offer a sense of protectiveness that would counteract some of the neglect of her early experiences. I hoped to meet the patient's overall emotional need to possess an interpersonal narrative for basic safety and trust.

I should note here that, although I spoke hypnotically, was no need for a formal induction. Patients with

Multiple Personality Disorder are highly suggestible. One only requires the patient's permission to proceed.)

The following is an excerpt from Beth's story, which in its entirety (and over many sessions), described a safe place with constant and protective spirits, and cycled through all times of the day, and all seasons of the year. I began and ended with our relationship in present time, but left the story itself open to whatever degree of identification she chose to bring to it. Here is an example.

"I'm going to tell a once-upon-a-time story about a little girl and the wonderful house she lives in. Of course, the little girl could be Beth, who—once she hears this story—can also have a wonderful house in a place in her thoughts where it will always be. The house goes on forever, if you wish, since the days and seasons in a child's life contain endless places for people and things, and for many thoughts and feelings to be. The house can wander off into as many hide-and-go-seek corridors as you can imagine, or it may simply be one warm and safe room just the right size for a small child.

"There is one more thing to say about this wonderful, safe house. No matter what room you are in, no matter where your fancy or the passage of time may take you, you will never be lonely. Every room, just as every door and window, is entrusted to the guardianship of a strong and peaceful spirit.

"The first room I would like Beth to know about is the room that is light with the gold of morning. In some ways, this is the special room for children, as it is filled with the light of the beginning of the day. This room has white curtains filtering the incoming rising light, which carries a soft breeze and brings the room into being. The light plays on white sheets and thrown-about colors of and blankets and teddy bears and rocking horses and dolls' houses. There are bird-sounds, and the feeling of the most comfortable bed mingled with good breakfast smells and morning conversation in the kitchen nearby. This is the room of the best morning ever, which will make every day look forward to the next.

"The spirit of this morning room is golden. She is as subtle as the light on the wall, or as beautiful and playful as a child garlanded with bright leaves and with her arms spilling over with toys. She is filled with inner laughter and her hands are eternally open. She is as calm as the moment before the sun rises, and light as the mist that touches the land and rivers at dawn. Her joyfulness rises from her knowledge that every morning is new, and her strength abides in the understanding that life renews itself forever.

"This first room is Beth's to linger in. When she wishes, she may move on to other rooms in the house. But this room will always provide the most cosy bed, the most satisfying awakening of all the rooms. This room makes it a pleasure to venture curiously into other rooms."

As the stories were told, Beth became more verbal and interactive, until one day, Elizabeth quietly told me: "I think Beth is integrating."

And so she was, merging into Elizabeth while reciting one of her favorite poems. There was a profound silence in the room, and I became aware of an almost tangible feeling of absence. And then the impression of absence was replaced by grief and finally resolution. Beth had united with Elizabeth, the host personality, bringing the trust needed to deepen the patient's belief in our relationship and r work.

When I was able to ask why Beth had integrated, Elizabeth simply explained: "She felt she had been acknowledged enough."

The assimilation of an awakening desire to trust had opened the book of Elizabeth's larger story. Through Beth, Elizabeth had found her way to the words—the voice—that unite patient and therapist and the world of relationship. From then on, Elizabeth was no longer mute, and the long process of building a narrative strong enough to support a healthy life was under way.

REFERENCES

References for Article: Uncovering "Forgotten" Child Abuse in the Psychotherapy of a Borderline Disorder of the Self

Breuer, J., & Freud, S. (1895). *Studies on hysteria.* (J. Strachey, Ed. and Trans.). New York: Basic Books, 1955.

Brown, D. P., & Fromm, E. (1986). *Hypnotherapy and hypnoanalysis.* Hillsdale, NJ: Erlbaum.

Erickson, M. H. (1966). The interspersal technique for symptom correction and pain control. *American Journal of Clinical Hypnosis, 3,* 198-209.

Masterson, J. F. (1976). *Psychotherapy of the borderline adult.* New York: Brunner/Mazel.

Watzlawick, P. (1978). *The language of change: Elements of therapeutic communication.* New York: Basic Books.

References for: Disorder of the Self, Trauma and the Use of Hypnosis

Bion, W. R. (1963). Elements of psycho-analysis. In Seven servants: four works by Wilfred R. Bion. New York: Jason Aronson, 1911.

Erickson, M.H., & Rossi, L. R. (1989). The February ma evolving consciousness and identity in hypnothe New York: Brunner/Mazel.

Erikson, E. H. (1950). Childhood and society. New York: W. W. Norton.

Janet, P. (1911). L'etat mental des hysteriques. Paris: Alcan. (Quoted by van der Kolk, et al. [1996], in Traumatic stress: the effects of overwhelming experience on mind, body and society. New York: Guilford Press.)

References for: Trauma in Personality Disorder — A Clinician's Handbook

American Psychiatric Association (1994). *DSM-IV: Diagnostic and statistical manual of mental disorders* 4th Ed. Washington, D.C.: American Psychiatric Association.

Blanck, G., & Blanck, R. (1974). *Ego psychology: Theory and practice.* New York: Columbia University Press.

Bowlby, J. (1988). Developmental psychiatry comes of age. *American Journal of Psychiatry,* 145: 1, 4.

Braun, B. (1986). Issues in the psychotherapy of multiple personality disorder. In *Treatment of multiple personality disorder,* B. Braun, (Ed.). Washington, D.C.: American Psychiatric Press.

Breuer, J., & Freud, S. (1895). *Studies on hysteria.* J. Strachey, (Ed.). New York: Basic Books.

Brown, D. (1997). Effective trauma treatment in the era of the false memory debate: The standard of science, the standard of care, and reducing malpractice liability. Lecture sponsored by the New Jersey Society for the Study of Dissociation. South Iselin, New Jersey.

~own, D., Scheflin A.W., & Hammond D.C., (1998). *Memory, trauma treatment & the law.* New York: Basic ~oks.

Fenichel, O. (1945). *The psychoanalytic theory of neurosis.* New York: W.W. Norton.

Freud, A. (1966). *The ego and the mechanisms of defense, Rev. Ed.* New York: International Universities Press.

Freud, S. (1908). Character and anal eroticism. In *Collected papers, Vol. 2*, E. Jones (Ed.). New York: Basic Books, 1959.

Freud, S. (1910). The future prospects of psychoanalytic therapy. In *Collected papers, Vol.2*, E. Jones (Ed.). New York: Basic Books, 1959.

Freud, S. (1912). The dynamics of the transference. In *Collected papers, Vol. 2*, E. Jones, (Ed.). New York: Basic Books, 1959.

Freud, S. (1914). Further recommendations in the technique of psychoanalysis. in *Collected papers, Vol.2*, E. Jones (Ed.). New York: Basic Books, 1959.

Freud, S. (1915). Some character-types met with in psychoanalytic work. In *Collected papers, Vol. 4*. E. Jones (Ed.). New York: Basic Books, 1959.

Giovacchini, P. (1979). Countertransference with primitive mental states. In *Countertransference*, L. Epstein & A. Feiner (Eds.). New York: Jason Aronson.

Guidelines for treating dissociative identity disorder (2000). *Journal of Trauma and Dissociation*, Herman, J. (1992). *Trauma and recovery.* New York: Basic Books.

Horowitz, M. (1997). *Stress response symptoms: PT5D, grief, and adjustment disorders.* Northvale, New York: Jason Aronson.

Klein, R. (1993). Schizoid personality disorder. In *The emerging self*, J. F. Masterson. New York: Brunner / Mazel.

Klein, R. (1995). Developmental theory. In *Disorders of the self: New therapeutic horizons*. J.F. Masterson & R. Klein (Eds.). New York: Brunner/Mazel.

Kluft, R. (1988). The postunification treatment of multiple personality disorder. *American Journal of Psychotherapy, LXII*, 2.

Langs, R.(1976). *The bipersonal field*. New York: Jason Aronson.

Laplanche, J., & Pontalis, J.B. (1973). *The language of psycho-analysis*. New York: W.W. Norton.

Mahler, M. (1972). Rapprochement subphase of the separation-individuation process. In *Selected papers of Margaret Mahler, Vol.* 2. New York: Jason Aronson, 1979.

Masterson, J.F. (1976). *Psychotherapy of the borderline adult*. New York: Brunner/Mazel.

Masterson, J.F. (1981). *The narcissistic and borderline disorders*. New York: Brunner/Mazel.

Masterson, J.F. (1985). *The real self*. New York: Brunner/Mazel.

Masterson, J.F. (1993). *The emerging self*. New York: Brunner/Mazel.

Orcutt, C. (1995). Integration of multiple personality disorder in the context of the Masterson Approach. In *Disorders of the self: New therapeutic horizons*. New York: Brunner/Mazel.

Orcutt, C. (1996). How do you dance when the music is stuck? The Masterson Approach to pre-Oedipal acting out. In *Issues in Psychoanalytic Psychology, 18:2*.

Putnam, F. (1989). *Diagnosis and treatment of multiple personality disorder*. New York: Guilford Press.

~h, W. (1949). *Character-analysis*. New York: Farrar, ~raus & Giroux.

Schore, A. (1999). The effect of psychological trauma on the developing brain. Lecture sponsored by The Masterson Institute for Psychoanalytic Psychotherapy. New York City.

Searles, H. (1979). The analyst's experience with jealousy. In *Countertransference,* L. Epstein & A. Feiner (Eds.). New York: Jason Aronson.

Spitz, R.A. (1965). *The first year of life: A psychoanalytic study of normal and deviant development of object relations.* New York: International University Press.

Spotnitz, H. (1979). Narcissistic countertransference. In *Countertransference,* L. Epstein & A. Feiner (Eds.). New York: Jason Aronson.

Van der Kolk, B.(1996). The complexity of adaptation to trauma: self-regulation, stimulus descrimination, and character development. In *Traumatic stress: the effects* of *overwhelming experience on mind, body, and society.* B. van der Kolk, A.C. McFarlane, & L. Weissaeth (Eds.). New York: Guilford.

Van der Kolk, B., Weissaeth, L., & van der Hart, O. (1996). History of trauma in psychiatry. In *Traumatic stress: the effects* of *overwhelming experience on mind, body, and society.* B. van der Kolk, A.C. McFarlane, & L. Weissaeth (Eds.). New York: Guilford.

Wilson, J. (1989). *Trauma, transformation and healing: an integrated approach to theory, research, and post-traumatic therapy.* New York: Brunner/Mazel.

Winnicott, D. W. (1960). The theory of parent-infant relationship. In *The maturational processes and the facilitating environment: Studies in the theory of emotional development.* New York: International Universities Press, 1965.